EDGAR CAYCE
ON
REJUVENATION
OF THE BODY

Edgar Cayce

on

Rejuvenation
of the Body

by John Van Auken

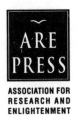

ARE
PRESS

ASSOCIATION FOR
RESEARCH AND
ENLIGHTENMENT

A.R.E. Press • Virginia Beach • Virginia

A.R.E. Press
215 67th Street
Virginia Beach, VA 23451-2061

Van Auken, John, 1946-
    Edgar Cayce's approach to rejuvenation of the body
/ by John Van Auken and the editors of the A.R.E.
        p.   cm.
    Originally published: Virginia Beach, Va. : Inner Vision Pub., 1995.
    ISBN 0-87604-359-7
    1. Cayce, Edgar, 1877-1945—Contributions in rejuvenation. 2. Rejuvenation—Psychological aspects. 3. Mental healing. 4. Mind and body therapies. I. Association for Research and Enlightenment. II. Title.
RZ401.V28   1996
613—dc20   96-3217

Cover Design by Richard Boyle

Contents

List of Illustrations

Introduction

Edgar Cayce has been called the "father of holistic medicine." In many ways this title fits him. In the early decades of this century he spoke on the virtues of working with the whole patient rather than some portion that seemed broken or diseased. He also believed that the mind, soul, and spirit of a person had to be taken into consideration when working on his or her body.

His work spanned nearly four decades, from the early 1900s to 1945. It is recorded and indexed by the association that he founded in 1931, the Association for Research and Enlightenment, Inc., or A.R.E. Basically, his discourses on various health topics were dictated to his longtime secretary, who took them down in shorthand and later typed them. They were eventually put on computer for easier access. There are over 14,000 of these discourses.

For this book I have focused on the ones dealing with rejuvenation of the human body. I have always believed that the body can rejuvenate itself; in fact, I believe it can do so indefinitely. Edgar Cayce was one of the few people I've come across who also believed this, and he had a great number of very specific things to say about this process. The more I studied his material, the more I liked it. In applying some of his ideas in my own life, I found that his concepts and methods really worked. Of course, time will be the ultimate tester of this, won't it?

I must warn you that his style of language is archaic, even by the standards of his time. But I have tried to edit his discourses in such a way as to retain the original meaning but deliver it in a more understandable manner. Nevertheless, the "thees" and "thous" remain to give you the true flavor of the man's comments. His secretary would often try to help by adding comments or words in [brackets], which I've left. She would also capitalize words he said with unusual emphasis. Normal emphasis she indicated by underlining, which I've put in bold typeface. For ease of identification, all his comments and his readings have been put within quotation marks.

Cayce was not a pontificator, but rather a quiet man who at a young age discovered that he could go into an unconscious state and retrieve information of all kinds. Strange as this may sound, I think you'll agree with me that his information on rejuvenation is sound and has a great deal of practical applicability.

Chapter 1

THE FUNDAMENTAL PRINCIPLES

When I first came across Edgar Cayce's material on health and the destiny of the body, I was amazed and excited. As a boy, I had heard preachers speak of eternal life and miracles of healing, but I had never realized how natural it could be until I read this material. Edgar Cayce presents a vision of what he calls "continual life," life that continues because it is *naturally one with the forces of Nature*. This life is in balance. It cooperates with the great forces of Life, not striving against them. When a body and mind are in cooperation and coordination with natural forces of the body, not in contention and willfulness, there is a rhythm that runs smoothly, nourishing and rejuvenating without end. In the Cayce approach, the best way to overcome death, illness or disease is to *preserve* a balanced, coordinated condition in the body and mind, with an attunement to the spiritual influence.

If the body has developed or inherited problems, then Cayce approaches it with an attitude of regeneration, resuscitation, and *rejuvenation*. There are no limitations, save those we put upon ourselves and the forces of God. For Cayce, the life force is that we call "spirit." Spirit is the *élan vital*, the kundalini, the glow of life—that which makes one virile, or the lack of it makes one lifeless and weak. Let's examine some of Cayce's key discourses.

THE BODY CAN REPRODUCE ITSELF

"The physical organism is constructed in such a way and manner that if the balance is kept in the diet, in the normal activity, and the mental forces replenished, then the body should readjust itself, refacilitate itself; making for not only resuscitation and revivifying of the necessary influences but carrying on and reproducing itself." 1040-1

"The body should in its elements be able, as it does continually, to reproduce itself; making for not only revivifying or resuscitating forces but keeping nominally alive." 1038-1

Notice his use of the word "nominal." In Cayce's vision life is much more than living healthfully. He often said, "It is not all of life to live nor all of death to die." Life must be lived for something, not just lived. Even when life is healthy, it is simply "nominal" until it has a purpose.

In most cases the Cayce discourses were generated by a question-and-answer format, as we see in this next dialogue:

"Q: Is it possible for our bodies to be rejuvenated in this incarnation?
"A: Possible. The body is an atomic structure, the units of energy around which there are the movements of atomic forces that are ever the pattern of a universe. Then, when these atoms are made to conform or rely upon

or to be one with the spiritual import, the spiritual activity, then they revivify, then they make for constructive forces." 262-85

Being "one with the spiritual import" is key to Cayce's method toward revivifying and making for constructive forces. This is a difficult concept for most of us to understand. As we continue, I believe we'll understand further.

"If there will be gained that consciousness, there need not be ever the necessity of a physical organism aging . . . seeing this, feeling this, knowing this, ye will find that not only does the body become revivified, but by creating in every atom of its being the knowledge of the activity of this Creative Force . . . spirit, mind, body are renewed." 1299-1

Notice his phrasing, "that consciousness" which will ultimately lead to no aging. What is that consciousness that he is referring to? Look at this next statement: (bold is author emphasis)

"In the present there may be gained within self the raising within self **that consciousness** of the at-onement with the spiritual forces that may revivify, regenerate, arouse that of health and happiness even under adverse conditions in materiality." 618-3

There is a state of consciousness that can heal. This consciousness is at-one with the spiritual forces. Cayce includes spiritual powers with mental and physical powers.

Notice this next comment which seems to be referring to an unknown sequence that leads to full, healthy life through some mystical path of transcendence.

"How is the way shown by the Master? What is the promise in Him? The last to be overcome is death. Death of what? The soul cannot die, for it is of God. The body may be revivified, rejuvenated—and it is to that end it may, the body, TRANSCEND the earth and its influences." 262-85

The last to be overcome is death? Are we on some sequence of life tests that ultimately lead to eternal life, as the religions have held? It seems that Cayce is confirming this, while also identifying many truths and practices that science holds to be critical to healthy life.

Since Cayce's discourses were given while he was in an altered state of consciousness (something like a deep hypnotic or meditative state), his metaphysical concepts reflect his process. He would lay his body down, focus his mind, and then through a series of changes—which included a shift in breathing, rapid eye movement, and striking imagery—he would attune himself to the spiritual forces, or as he often put it "the Universal Consciousness of God."

(Note: Most of his discourses were recorded by shorthand, only a few are on voice recording equipment. Therefore, the stenographer made a practice of capitalizing all words that were spoken loudly or with unusual emphasis, while slight emphasis was underlined. In this book, I've left the all-capitalized words, but changed the underlined words to bold. See the Introduction for further insight into the process and language of Cayce discourses.)

If we accept the principles in his discourses, then health and a long life are a matter of applying some specific principles along with some therapeutic applications in our bodies, minds, and spirits. For Cayce, all three of these aspects of our being have to be in cooperation and full activity before true healing and rejuvenation can take hold.

A HOLISTIC APPROACH

The Cayce approach is a holistic approach. As we will see in later sections, one must take into consideration all subsystems of the body-system, as well as the other aspects of the being—mind and spirit. Within the body, Cayce strives for *overall* improvement, in a *balanced* and *coordinated* manner, never focusing on just one portion of the system, but seeing the system as just that, a system! And, one must work on the mind and soul, as well as the body—perhaps, more than the body.

Beyond the body, Cayce insists that true healing and wellness must *include* the condition and activity of the mind, as well as the purposes and hopes of the spirit. Each of us is first a spiritual being, with mental powers and activities, which is incarnate in a physical body. Therefore, use of the mental and spiritual forces is as important as one's use of the physical.

"Bringing normalcy and a revivifying of purposes, desires or ambitions—the body WHOLE must be taken into consideration; that is, the physical, the mental and the spiritual attributes of the body." 1189-2

"Keep the mental and the spiritual forces **active** during the [therapeutic] applications; not done as rote! Know within self something is being accomplished through the [therapeutic] applications." 1158-1

This was a frequent instruction from Cayce: "See, feel, know something is being accomplished." Nothing is more powerful than the mindful presence of faith and belief and expectancy. For Cayce, and many other healers, the mind is a powerful player in the process of healing.

"To be sure, as it has been indicated again and again, there is that within the physical forces of the body which may be revivified or rejuvenated, if it is kept in a constructive way and manner. This requires, necessarily, the proper thinking, the proper living, the proper application of those influences in the experience of an entity in its associations with everything about a body." 681-2

HEALING & HEALTH COME FROM WITHIN

For Cayce, the healing of illness and the maintenance of health is a result of a coordination of body-mind-spirit, and this begins *within* us. As most doctors confess, the ultimate decision for life or death is within the individual. One can apply all the miracles of modern science or mystical religion, but unless something within that person is stirred to live, to rejuvenate, little can be accomplished.

This is perhaps the most difficult concept for us to grasp. Despite the applications of medicines, hi-tech machines, foods, and physical manipulations, the body actually receives its ultimate healing and wellness from the unseen forces within it. All these other elements are simply catalysts or stimulants to encourage the body forces to bring about the healthy condition.

"From whence comes the healing? Whether there is administered a drug, a correcting or an adjustment of a subluxation, or the alleviating of a strain upon the muscles, or the revivifying through electrical forces; they are ONE, and the healing comes from WITHIN! Not by the method does the healing come, though the consciousness of the individual IS such that this or that method IS the one that is more effective in the individual case in **arousing the forces from within**. But the METHODS are NOT ideals. The IDEAL must be kept in the proper SOURCE." 969-1

Here Cayce is commenting on the truth that the method is not the miracle. Yet, he acknowledges that method is critical because of the belief system. The mind-set of the individual must be considered when deciding on what method to use. As Cayce once noted, "You cannot cure a quinine mind of malaria with anything but quinine!" Nevertheless, it is not the quinine that is the healer, but the mind within the person who believes the quinine will heal. The source of healing is within us.

If we realize this, and begin to take hold of our inner thoughts, beliefs, and consciousness, then we can make significant changes in our outer condition.

We've already seen the first of the next two excerpts, but let's look at it again, this time with the emphasis on the "within."

"In the present there may be gained within self the raising **within** self that consciousness of the at-onement with the spiritual forces that may revivify, regenerate, arouse that of health and happiness even under adverse conditions in materiality." 618-3

"The revivifying forces are the NATURAL sources of energies through quietness **within** any given activity that makes for strengthening for resistances of every nature in a physical body." 587-5

In this next discourse you'll notice a reference to "thine inner self." When I first came across it, I was curious about this other self that I was not familiar with, especially since Cayce frequently indicated that it was quite distinct from my outer self. Then, one day, while waking from a dream I had an experience that helped me sense the difference between my outer and inner self. I was dreaming. I knew I was dreaming, and I was enjoying the dream and thinking about how I would record this dream in my dream journal when I finally awoke. When I did fully wake up, I remembered the dream and my desire to record it, but I decided to first go to the bathroom and empty my bladder. When I returned, I had absolutely no recall of the dream. Nothing! I couldn't believe it. There was no dream content in my mind. Therefore, I lay back down on the bed and began to go back into sleep, when suddenly there was the dream content. In my desire to understand this, I practiced moving from the dream state out into the conscious state to see if I could better bridge these two realities. It became clear to me that when I was in the dream, I really felt like "I" was conscious and dreaming. However, when I was out in the conscious state, I also felt that "I" was conscious, but without any dream content. The more I played with this movement between the two realities, the more I realized that there truly were two, clearly discernible parts to my being. One was aligned with my subconscious mind, and experienced and possessed the dream content. And the other was aligned with my conscious mind and physical world and contained no dream unless I gradually awoke and purposefully conveyed the content matter over to it, and even then I could barely hold onto it for any length of time! Despite these two distinct parts of me, I felt that I was really me when I was in either of the two aspects of myself. "I" was dreaming, and "I" was emptying my bladder. My inner and outer self were familiar to me, but not to each other. The veil between them was so opaque that I could not see back into the subconscious once I was fully in the outer consciousness. But the movement between the two was so subtle that I didn't even notice I had moved out of one and into the other.

In this next discourse we have Cayce referring to the work or role our inner self plays in the healing process, and the help it needs.

"The revivifying influences will give thine inner self that which will create, that which will build in the body, as thou holdest to that thou knowest **within** thine self—that He, the Giver of all good and perfect gifts, is renewing thy strength and thy life **within** thee; and that thou wilt USE same in His service so long as the days are given unto thee for thy activities in this material world. And we will find STRENGTH being built in thine body as the stamina of steel! And, as the vital forces renew thy vitality in thine body, USE thy mental self." 716-2

If we also remember that the subconscious mind (the mind of the inner self) is amenable to suggestion, then many of Cayce's guidelines about positive belief and active mindfulness make real sense.

Coordinating body-mind-spirit and taking hold of the forces within us will lead us to health and rejuvenation. However, for Cayce, the answer to why we want to be healthy and rejuvenated is as important as how we achieve it.

THE RIGHT IDEAL & PURPOSE

If we came to Cayce for guidance, he would not first tell us to pray, meditate or seek a dream; he'd tell us to set an ideal, a standard by which we could measure the value of whatever we do. The ideal is like a pole star by which we guide our lives and decisions. Rather than letting the circumstances of life rule us, we set the direction, the purpose and the ultimate condition sought; then everything moves toward realizing that. Even when circumstances are hard against us, we, like the captain of a great sailing ship, tack against that wind, ever moving toward our ideal—and when the wind eases up or changes direction, we'll be in a better position than if we had simply let the circumstances (the winds) of life take us wherever they would lead.

This is the power of an ideal. It helps us understand *why* we are doing something, *what* we are desiring to realize or be, and gives us a *measuring rod* by which to judge the elements of a life-decision and thereby make decisions based on our *inner* desire rather than the outer world's forces.

"Put thy ideal in those things that bespeak of the continuity of life; the regeneration of the spiritual body, the revivifying of the temporal body for SPIRITUAL purposes, that the seed may go forth even as the Teacher gave, 'Sin no more, but present thy body as a living sacrifice; holy, acceptable unto Him, for it is a reasonable service.' " 969-1

"Begin to PLAN as to what the body will DO when and AS the improvements come. Not only be good, be good FOR SOMETHING! Hold to that which is Truth!" 572-5

"These bespeak of something innate within self that bespeaks of the abilities of the soul, mind and body to revivify and rejuvenate itself as to an ideal." 578-2

Two people can do exactly the same things toward rejuvenation and wellness, but get different results. So often, the influencing force in these cases is their attitude. One is hopeful and expectant, the other doubts or feels unworthy. Attitude is a powerful, unseen influence in the outcome of any activity.

"To be sure, there should be rather that expectant attitude of the body ... for unless there is the expectancy, unless there is hope, the mind's outlook becomes a drag, a drug on one that is being attacked from within by the various diseases of a physical body." 572-5

Cayce often hyphenated the word *disease* in an effort to convey the real source of disease as being a dis-ease in the system, physically and mentally. When a being is at ease with itself, health is usually present. But health cannot be maintained long when something within a person is uneasy, or at *dis-ease*. Notice also how he continues to emphasize the importance of the right mental attitude: being hopeful and expectant.

Doubt was also on Cayce's list of "don'ts," as we see in this next instruction:

"DO NOT become morose. Do not doubt the abilities of those influences in the spiritual life to meet the needs of the body physically, mentally, spiritually, and we will revivify these things." 458-2

"Nothing save self stands in the way of the entity MAKING or becoming a channel of blessings to many! For the entity may be assured, for the entity will find, **nothing** in heaven or hell or earth may separate thee from the knowledge and the use of the I AM PRESENCE within, save selfishness—or self!" 440-20

This is a hard one to accept. Few of us take full responsibility for our circumstances in life and in health. But it sure appears that Cayce is listing "self" as the only limitation to success.

This next Cayce comment reminds me of my parents' admonitions to "pull yourself together" or "get hold of yourself." Mind over circumstances, whether they are physical, emotional or mental, is a powerful tool toward changing the prevailing condition. But Cayce even takes this a step further, saying that we shouldn't even use discouraging remarks when we are struggling to overcome a condition.

> "Hence mind over matter is not to be lightly spoken of, nor is there any disparaging remark to be made as to the ability of the body-physical to be revivified, resuscitated, spiritualized such that there is no reaction that may not be revivified." 1152-5

The Cayce records are filled with the admonition to "live what you know to be true and right." Our actions must reflect our deepest beliefs and values. If they do, then the Life Force can flow through us without getting meshed in a web of hypocrisy, contradiction, and disharmony. He often identified incoordination of the two nervous systems as one of the major causes of illness, equating it with the two parts of ourselves (inner and outer) being at war with one another. Here he calls for us to hold to a simple truth:

> "For HE hath shown the way—not by some mysterious fluid, not by some unusual vibration, but by the simple method of LIVING that which is LIFE itself. THINK no evil; HEAR no

evil. And as the Truth flows as a stream of life through the Mind in all its phases or aspects, and purifies same, so will it purify and revivify and rejuvenate the body. For once this effacement urge is overcome, then may there begin the rejuvenation." 294-183

In this case, and with many of us today, we actually seem to get in a self-destructive mode, or as Cayce said, an "effacement urge." Who can save us from ourselves? All the outer applications can't overcome the desires of the ruler of the house. First, one must stop effacing oneself or destroying oneself, for whatever reason we may think justified. Then, self can be transformed.

"Mind IS the master." 2529-1

Paradoxically, this powerful statement is frequently offset by a "nevertheless" statement, such as this one:

"Yet, physical conditions need the [therapeutic] activity that may regenerate or revivify the abilities for reproduction of self through the afflicted or disturbed areas of the body." 2529-1

One can only conclude that the mind is the master, yet we also need therapeutic applications to help along the regenerative process.

"It may appear long, but—keep that attitude of being the channel through which more love of the divine nature may be given, even as ye would be SHOWN that towards the ways and manners for the helpfulness in the material physical body." 1199-3

Cayce often encouraged those who were in the

worst situations to get out of their self-absorbtion with their problems by simply looking around for someone else who needed help, and helping them— with no thought of reward. Something in the spirit of helpfulness has a magical effect upon the helper.

In this next case we see someone who is suppressing herself, either from guilt, self-consciousness, anxiety, or fear. Since every living thing has an inner drive to express life, suppression is against the flow of life, and must therefore be transformed in order for life to flow and health to return. He encourages her to get interested in something, as well as keeping up with the therapy.

"The destruction of the blood forces [is] by SUPPRESSION of self in a mental manner. Hence, the necessity of directing and interesting self in a FAD, or even a FANCY, and keeping self interested in same, as well as correcting the physical conditions." 5554-2

As we have seen, the mind and the mental attitude play major roles in the healing and health maintenance process.

Finally, Cayce gives the best attitude to hold for maintaining youth and youthful influences:

"Let age only ripen thee. For one is ever as young as the heart and the purpose. Keep sweet. Keep friendly. Keep loving, if ye would keep young." 3420-1

THE SEVEN-YEAR CYCLE OF RENEWAL

According to the Cayce material, the body rebuilds itself in its entirety (every cell) every seven years. Therefore, no matter what problem we have, if we would apply ourselves to changing it, and work

patiently throughout the seven-year cycle, our bodies would have rebuilt every cell according to this
new ideal, this new goal, this new hope.

"Every seven years there is performed an
entire renewal of the whole structural or ana-
tomical body." 887-4

"In this particular body . . . the system will
produce that which will enable the body to
continue without any letdown for a period of
another cycle to three cycles. Then, before
there is any real letdown in the abilities of the
body, there should be at least twenty-one more
years of activity." [7 years per cycle, times 3
cycles, equals 21 years] (This person was an
adult, but their age at the time of these comments was unkown.) 1064-1

I have consciously gone through four seven-year
cycles using Cayce's concepts, diet, and practices. I
can attest to its powerful influence on transforming
bodily, attitudinal and emotional habits and conditions into new, healthier states of being. And, with
this cycle in mind, I can take whatever I am now,
and apply myself toward changing that over the
next seven years. You must understand, that for
Cayce, each cell of our body has its consciousness,
and that consciousness can be raised or lowered.
Therefore, if every cell is changed every seven years,
then everything and anything can be changed!
The seven-year cycle is an important concept to
keep in mind as we work toward healing and health
maintenance.

ATTUNEMENT IS REQUIRED

Unique to Cayce's vision is the idea that seekers
of healing and health must *attune* themselves to the

Divine within every cell of their bodies in order to fully realize the perfected condition. It's like a pattern, a code, a vibration that possesses life in its *ideal* condition—continual and healthy life—and when we attune to it, we begin to imbue ourselves with this perfected life pattern or state of being.

"It will require that there be such an attitude in mind, in purpose, in hope, and in relationships to others, that each cell of the body may be **atttuned to the Divine within.** Each cell must become expectant, that there may be the renewing, the revivifying of the relationships that the soul-entity bears to Creative Forces." 3511-1 (bold is author emphasis)

"Thus there may be a revivifying, a resuscitating, a creating of an environment such that the body-mind, with its **spiritual** concepts and its **spiritual** understanding, may arouse the whole of the body-forces to their better functionings." 1620-1 (bold is author emphasis)

"For the body mentally, in its spiritual attributes for the physical self, may hold much in this manner—as the applications are made, osteopathically, electrically—not for things to be gotten through with, but SEE, FEEL, KNOW that these are channels and measures through which **the divine may operate** for effective activity in this body!" 1299-1 (bold is author emphasis)

In this next case we see that some problems are so big, so deep, so painfully possessing that we need divine help to fully overcome their influence upon us.

"The addition of energy-building forces has not removed the hurt, the disappointment. For this has attacked the physical body through the sensory and sympathetic nervous system, causing the reaction. Not that there is any mental disturbance, no. It is rather a hurt, an injury, a disappointment such that there can only come the renewing, the revivifying, by putting the whole trust, faith and renewed life **in Divine hands.**" 4037-1 (bold is author emphasis)

"Being able to raise within the vibrations of individuals to that which is a resuscitating, a revivifying influence and force **through the deep meditation** (the attunement of self to the higher vibrations in Creative Forces), these are manifested in man through the promises that are coming from Creative Forces or Energy itself!" 993-4 (bold is author emphasis but Cayce's parenthetical comment)

Meditation, especially deep meditation, is one of the most commonly recommended practices in the Edgar Cayce work. For him, meditation was necessary in order for humans to bridge the gap between this world of outer, physical consciousness and the inner world of the subconscious, soul and spirit forces. In this particular discourse, he is identifying the deep meditation practice as a means to attuning self "to the higher vibrations in Creative Forces." *Creative Forces* is a Cayce term for those forces many of us associate with God, Nature and the powers of Life itself—or as he says himself "Energy itself!" Learning to become outwardly still and quiet, while awakening inwardly to the deeper vibrations, especially those with a spiritual quality to them, can result in higher vibes and the flow of energy, resuscitating energy, through our bodies, minds and souls. Because of this, I've included a chapter on meditation in this book.

Let's continue looking into attunement, especially attunement to the Divine within.

"Put hope and trust and faith in the Divine within—the revivifying, the rejuvenating of that spirit of life and truth within every atom of the body. This will put to flight all of those things that hinder a body from giving expression of the most hopeful, the most beautiful." 572-5

"There are those forces as may be had from the study, the analyzing of those truths presented in the light of HIS ministry—that One who is the way, the truth and the light. The **analyzing** of these, and the **application** of same in the lives of individuals is an individual experience. But the closer, the nearer one **applies** those tenets, those truths, those principles in one's daily experience, the greater is the ability of the mental and spiritual self to revivify the physical activities of any given body." 2074-1 (bold is author emphasis)

Again, we see Cayce driving hard on the principle of applying ourselves—seeking, studying, analyzing those tenets and principles we know to be of great importance to us, mentally and spiritually. As the great psychologist Carl Jung pointed out, we cannot deny that there is a spiritual component to humans, no matter how illogical it may appear to some of us. Spirit, and spiritual truths, are important to the overall health of humans, from the most primitive to the most sophisticated.

Overall, the Cayce material is universal in its spiritual content, including wisdom from all the great religions, especially those that teach there is one God and a brotherhood, sisterhood among humankind. However, there is an emphasis in the

Cayce material on Jesus Christ and His teachings and ministry. But it is a much bigger vision than most Christian religions acknowledge. This next excerpt takes us far beyond the boundaries that most of us think of for rejuvenation.

"When the Prince of Peace came into the earth for the completing of His OWN development in the earth, HE overcame the flesh AND temptation. So He became the first of those that overcame death in the body, enabling Him to so illuminate, to so revivify that body as to take it up again, even when those fluids of the body had been drained away by the nail holes in His hands and by the spear piercing His side." 1152-1

BALANCE & COORDINATION ARE REQUIRED

Balance and coordination are a part of Cayce's approach. Most often it was coordination of the two nervous systems, which we will look into later. It was balance throughout the system, rather than accentuation of one system over another. Here are a few examples of his comments:

"To be rejuvenated, the body must be kept in a condition of construction; to ever find that the heart, the digestive organs' combination of elimination and assimilation, the hair, the scalp, the nasal, the eye, the ear, the throat, the bronchi, the lungs, the structual forces of the body work as a UNIT, or as ONE! And then we may find, and do find, the body BUILDING, ever." 681-2

"There must be kept a body-balance." 681-2

"There is more than one manner of eliminating the conditions, but inasmuch as there needs to be the reviving, the revivifying and the **coordination** of the vibratory forces through the body—we find these as we will give would be the more preferable ways and manners for making for the corrections to be of a permanent nature; thus revivifying the **whole** of the body." 1196-1 (author emphasis)

"There may be created that balance of cooperation and **coordination** throughout the physical forces of the body, revivifying those disturbances to a constructive activity, rather than a tearing down; and creating those balances in the coordination of the mental with the spiritual for the material activity." 1173-8 (author emphasis)

"As there is the revivifying of the **whole system**, this [ailment] should take on a different condition, as the GENERAL condition is helped, see?" 366-3 (bold is author emphasis)

Cayce is going for an improvement in the "general" condition of the system, and that will in turn help the specific ailment be overcome. He often sought overall balance and coordination throughout the body rather than focused work on one part of the body.

Chapter 2

THE MECHANICS OF REJUVENATION

Cayce had much to say about certain subsystems of the human body, namely the blood, nerves, and glands.

THE BLOOD

In the whole of Cayce's work, the blood seems to be the single most important system for rejuvenation of the body. Clean, vitalized, ionized, ironized, and carbonized blood helps the body eliminate the forces that bring aging and death. This quality of blood also delivers the constructive, revivifying, and rejuvenating forces that bring life, and the extension of life. Here are some of those extracts:

"The body rebuilds itself CONSTANTLY, through what? The BLOOD supply!" 683-3

"In the blood supply of this body (as in most bodies, though it may be illustrated in the activities of the bloodstream more thoroughly here than in most physical bodies) lies the life and extenuation of life, the abilities to create and to eliminate from the system destructive forces, as well as within same create constructive, resuscitating, revivifying forces within the body." 443-2

"Gradually, as the strength and resistance and the bloodstream becomes renewed and revivified, the eliminations and the drosses become less and less a portion of the problem." 1173-1

RE-IONIZING THE BLOOD

"Q: Have I sufficient magnetism?
"A: This rises and falls easily, owing to the lack of ionization through the system. Hence the low electrical and vibratory form of activity necessary in the body." 1811-1

"This re-ionizing of the bloodstream, the revivifying of the flows to the internal as well as the external circulation, should revitalize these [weaknesses of the body]." 1299-1

"There must be kept a body-balance, then. Hence, ionizing of the energies from all the radial forces about the superficial circulation—as may be taken by the activities that come from electrical emanations about self—is helpful. But if these are passed as the equalizing from one extremity to another, and then the exercises, so much the better!" 681-2

This phrase, "passed . . . from one extremity to another" is a reference to Cayce's teachings about the positive benefits of the old spiritual practice of laying hands on other people to give to them this "electrical emanation" that can be transferred from one individual to another, especially if there is a love relationship and even more so if there is a genetic connection, such as parent to child. Every body has an electrical/magnetic energy within and about it. Of course this is the low, bio-electrical energy, not the type that is flowing through power lines on the street. If reasonably healthy people, with good intentions and some sense of what they are doing, lay their hands on another person, then the current (low, bio-current) can flow to that person, and the individual can use this energy. Cayce most often recommended this be done just before the recipient is going to sleep for the night.

Occasionally, Cayce recommended a battery-like device be used to help the body rebuild. Cayce likened the device to a radio, a device that helps "tune" the body to a certain frequency. This is why he initially called it a "radio-active appliance." It has absolutely nothing to do with nuclear radioactivity. Today, most of us refer to this appliance as the "radial appliance" to keep from confusing it with nuclear radioactivity. The appliance is described in a later section of this book.

"The use of the Radio-Active Appliance would RE-IONIZE the system, if this is used of evenings before retiring. Not AFTER retiring, but BEFORE retiring; while the body meditates use the Appliance." 189-4

"Each day we would use the Radio-Active Appliance for one hour, attached to opposite sides of the body; right wrist, left ankle; left wrist, right ankle. This is to create—by the body-vibrations, that are brought to activative forces of forcing through the whole of the circulatory forces that renewal of energy and vitality—re-ionizing of the vital forces.

"After the treatment with the Radio-Active Appliance each day we would use a massage with an equal combination of Olive Oil and Tincture of Myrrh; that this may stimulate the circulation.

"These do, and keep activities cheery. Thus we may bring the better conditions for the body." 1384-2

Occasionally, a body can be too ionized, as in this case:

"However, as we find, that needed instead of RE-ionizing is rather DE-ionizing of the vibratory forces of the body, for the better conditions." 1297-2

CARBON IN THE BLOOD

Here we see an unusual approach to revitalizing the blood.

"[We need] the active forces of carbon, or oxygen through the decomposed carbon, electrified, released IN the system—so as to re-VITALIZE the energies in the bloodstream." 5645-1

"The body needs rest, mentally and physically, and the outside, open air, plenty of carbon—oxygen for the system—so that the blood supply is re-ironized [re-ionized] throughout. Plenty of those food values that carry much of iron and iodine, reducing potashes in the system, as to relieve nerve tension." 5554-2

It appears that Cayce is using the word *carbon* in a manner similar to how we use *carbohydrate*. Later, in the section on Carbon Food, this will be explained more fully.

BLOOD AS WE KNOW IT TODAY

Today we have a much greater knowledge of blood and its function than they did in the 1920s and '30s. Let's look at blood and its role in the magnificent human body. This will help us understand how our bodies work, and specifically why Cayce put so much emphasis on the blood and its role in rejuvenation.

In our bodies are more than 60,000 *miles* of blood vessels! A single drop of blood goes through the entire body more than 1,000 times a day! It takes just about one minute for a drop of blood to go from our hearts to our toes and back again.

Blood cells are relatively small when compared with other cells in our bodies, such as liver cells. Some of the passages that the blood has to go through are so small that blood cells must go through one cell at a time in single file (i.e., through the capillaries).

Blood is actually rather complex, composed of several components. Blood cells are made mainly in bone marrow. Blood cells flow through the body in a yellowish liquid called plasma. Plasma also contains food, waste, salts, and other substances. Blood is composed of red and white blood cells and platelets.

RED BLOOD CELLS

Red blood cells are the most common cells in blood. A normal body creates red blood cells at the rate of 90-100 million a minute! Hemoglobin is the key ingredient in red blood cells. It gives them their red color and is the carrier for oxygen and carbon dioxide. These red cells carry oxygen from the lungs throughout the body giving life to each cell, while at the same time collecting carbon dioxide from the cells and delivering it to the lungs for discharge. A red blood cell lives for about four months. It will make roughly 170,000 journeys around the body in

THE BLOOD CIRCULATORY SYSTEM
Heart, 1. Arteries, and 2. Veins

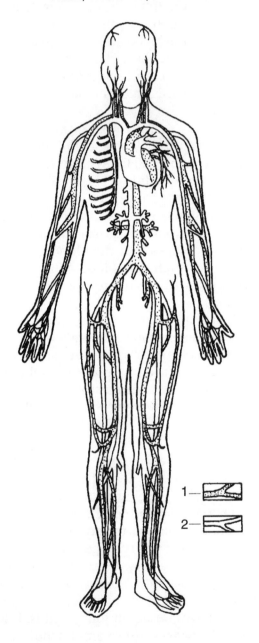

1 —

2 —

its lifetime. Perhaps this is why Cayce says that eventually we will learn how to interpret the condition of the whole body by examining a single drop of blood.

WHITE BLOOD CELLS

White blood cells are the protectors and warriors of the body. They are larger than red blood cells, live only for seven to fourteen days. There are many fewer white blood cells in the body than red, but the white cells can multiply extremely fast when the body needs their protective help. When an alien cell enters the body, such as a virus or bacteria, the white blood cells attack it. They can even change shape in order to surround the invader and protect nearby cells from its destructive influence. They can actually consume and digest the cell. If the white blood cells determine that the invasion is beyond their power to digest the invaders, they produce a powerful poison against that particular invader—an antibody. This creates an environment in which the invader cannot multiply and take a hold on the system. Once a specific poison or antibody is made, it stays in the system forever. A mother can actually give antibodies to her child through her breast milk and colostrum, thereby passing along protection to her child before his or her body even comes into contact with the virus or bacteria.

BLOOD PLATELETS

Platelets are more numerous than white blood cells. In a drop of blood there are approximately 250,000,000 red blood cells, 400,000 white blood cells and 15,000,000 platelets. The platelets are even smaller than the red blood cells. The platelets protect us from losing all our blood through a wound. As the blood pours through a wound, the platelets go into action. They become sticky and cling together, slowing the flow of blood. Eventually, they dry and form a crust or scab at the site of the wound, stopping the flow of blood.

The blood actually needs cleaning. It gets this through the lymph system and the kidneys.

THE LYMPH SYSTEM

Throughout our bodies is a network of clear, watery liquid called lymph. All along the system there are bean-sized lymph nodes where extra white blood cells gather to help clean the blood of impurities. A group of lymph nodes becomes a gland, such as the lymph glands along the side of our throats, under our arms and on the inside of our thighs. If we are sick, these glands often swell and become painful due to multiplication of white blood cells in the battle to overcome the germs' invasion. Lymph was very important in the Cayce approach. He encouraged exercise and massage to keep the lymph system operating at peak performance and drained of any drosses. Unlike the blood system, the lymph system has no pump to move its liquid along. It depends on the muscle movement of our bodies to move its fluid through the system. If we don't get enough exercise, then it slows or stops. Massage can help get it moving and empty its drosses.

Here's one of Cayce's insights into this:

"If a cell is left in the system that should be eliminated, or if it is of a condition of inactivity, then all the cells gathered about it cannot heal that cell. It [the system] **must** produce sufficient of the lymph or leukocyte [white blood cells] to move it out of the system, to let the new supply take its place! Just as a comparison, a rotten apple left in a barrel may make all of these rotten; yet no matter how many sound ones are put about it, the rotten one will never be made sound." 243-7

THE LYMPH SYSTEM

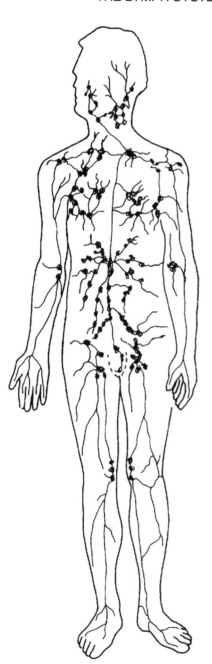

A circulating system of clear fluid that helps clean the blood and protect against illness. It relies on bodily movement to circulate its vital fluid. The darker areas are lymph nodes and glands.

THE KIDNEYS

Every day the blood supply flows through the kidneys hundreds of times. The water in the blood is squeezed out and filtered. Unwanted waste and poisons are removed. The main waste is urea (thus the term *urine*), which is produced during digestion of foods. Too much urea in the blood is poisonous to the body. Therefore, the kidneys filter urea from the blood. They also filter leftover vitamins, medicines, and alcohol. Most of the water is put back into the blood system, but some is transferred to the bladder for removal. This bladder water contains the wastes and poisons.

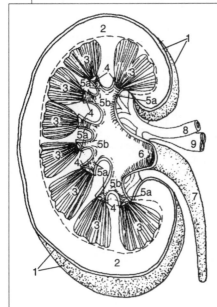

THE KIDNEY
The great filter of
the body

1.	Renal capsule	5b.	Major calyces
2.	Cortex	6.	Urine collector
3.	Medulla	7.	Urine tube to bladder
	(pyramid filters)	8.	Blood in
4.	Papilla	9.	Blood out
5a.	Minor calyces		

THE HEART & VESSELS

This brings us to the heart and its 60,000 miles of vessels. The heart is a very powerful muscle that pushes blood along thousands of miles of blood vessels. It has to do this in a regular, rhythmical manner and for many, many years. And when needed, it must beat at greater or lesser rates according to the mind's and body's demands. Throughout its vessel system are valves and controls to keep the flow even and going in the right direction, even if we stand on our hands. When the blood isn't flowing to some part of our body, we feel cold and prickly ("my leg's asleep"). The blood pressure in veins is less than the

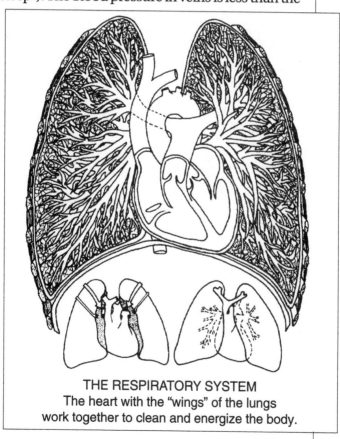

THE RESPIRATORY SYSTEM
The heart with the "wings" of the lungs
work together to clean and energize the body.

pressure in arteries because the blood leaves the heart to the arteries first, and by the time it reaches the veins much of its push-pressure is lost. Because of this, arteries are more elastic than veins.

THE LUNGS & LIVER

Blood flow to the lungs and liver is of great importance to our healthy survival. In the lungs the blood is cleansed of carbon dioxide and filled with oxygen. The oxygen is used in a process called respiration, where oxygen and nutrients are converted

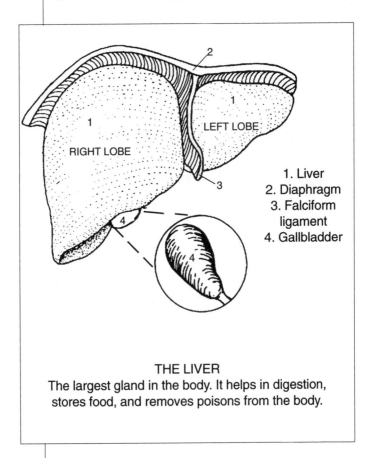

1. Liver
2. Diaphragm
3. Falciform ligament
4. Gallbladder

THE LIVER
The largest gland in the body. It helps in digestion, stores food, and removes poisons from the body.

into energy in the cells. The blood and liver relationship is more complex. The blood transports "foods" from the small intestines to the liver for storage for later use. Then, as needed, the liver can release these stored "foods" into the blood system to nourish cells throughout the body.

The blood and the blood system are one of the most important parts of the body. If rejuvenation is our goal, then we must make sure the blood is clean, oxygenated, nutrient-rich and flowing regularly and freely throughout our bodies. Thus, the cells of our bodies are nourished and cleaned, with no buildup of waste and poisons that ultimately destroys the cells. Enemies of the body are also controlled by strong, healthy blood and lymph, keeping the body healthy and free of disease.

THE NERVES

In addition to revitalizing the blood, Cayce frequently instructed health-seekers to revitalize the nervous system. The nervous system is a chemical-electrical system. Cayce identifies electrical forces with God and the Life or Creative Force.

"As the electrical vibrations are given, know that Life itself, to be sure, is the Creative Force or God, yet its manifestions in man are electrical, or vibratory. Know then that the force in nature that is called electrical or electricity is that same force ye worship as Creative or God in action!

"Seeing this, feeling this, knowing this, ye will find that not only does the body become revivified, but by the creating in every atom of its being the knowledge of the activity of this Creative Force or Principle as related to spirit, mind, body, all three are **renewed**." 1299-1

"We find the nerve system overtaxed and the body assimilating fear rather than stimulus of the nature to give relief to the body." 4790-1

Too often we see people or become people who are too nervous, fearful, anxious or strained. This does not allow the body sufficient energy and rest to rejuvenate. A good, sound nervous system is important for true, deep healing and rejuvenation.

We find Cayce approaching the nervous system in the same manner he approached the blood system.

RE-IONIZING NERVE FORCES

"We find that there is the lack of ionization of the nerve forces, owing to the great strain that has been put upon the whole of the nervous system, as well as the manner of the circulatory system. Yet, these may be aided in creating a better coordination between the superficial and deeper circulation, and a better reaction or activity through the assimilating forces of the body." 1553-1

Apparently, re-ionizing without coordination does little to help, as we see in this next answer:

"Q: Would breathing exercise for re-ionizing the system together with the head-and-neck exercise be well at this time?

"A: Not until we get the body coordinating better physically and physically-mentally. Then these exercises would be very well." 1523-17

Cayce's phrase "physically-mentally" is often his way of addressing the nervous system. It is the system that connects body and mind. According to

Cayce and many other people in the healing arts, the mind's disposition affects the body's condition, and the nervous system is their meeting place.

Again, he would recommend the radio-active appliance or radial appliance to help with this process. As we will see in a later chapter, he claimed that the appliance would help the attitudes and moods as well as the electrical forces. Here are a few more of these extracts to give you a sample of his comments on electrical vibrations and their influence.

"The electric forces [will] re-ionize the body-vitality. This would be of the low forms of electrical vibration as from the low static vibratory influence, rather than the direct currents." 1472-8

"[We need] re-ionizing or re-vitalizing or re-charging—as it were—the whole vital forces of the body itself . . . to bring much better and much nearer NORMAL coordination." 1038-1

"Use those vibrations as may be set up by the Radio-Active Appliance as may be attached to the body for the attuning or ionizing or re-electrifying of the energies of the system." 1125-2

CARBONIZING NERVE FORCES

In this next reading, we get a clear view into Cayce's perspective on the nervous system's role in the human body and its components.

"The body itself, the whole body, is not in as good condition to rebuild as we have had before, because we find the carbon of the body, or the storage battery of the body, **which we have of course in the nerve tissue in the gray**

THE NERVOUS SYSTEM
1. Brain
2. Nerve network

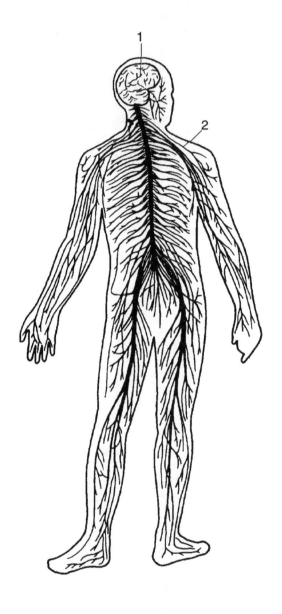

THE NERVOUS SYSTEM
3. Voluntary muscles
4. Involuntary organs (includes skin)

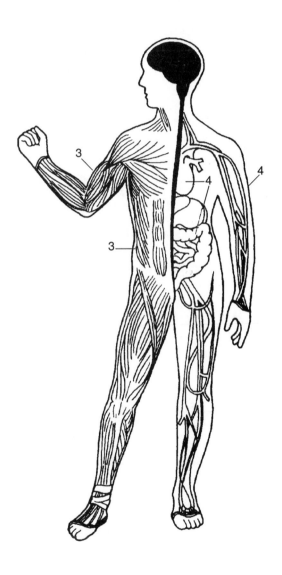

THE NERVE CELLS
Chemical-electric receivers and transmitters.

1. Dendrite
2. Nucleus
3. Cell body
4. Axis cylinder
5. Node of Ranvier
6. Myelin sheath

7. Sheath of Schwann's cell
8. Nucleus of Schwann's cell
9. Terminal branches
10. Pre-synaptic membrane
11. Post-synaptic membrane
12. Synaptic cleft

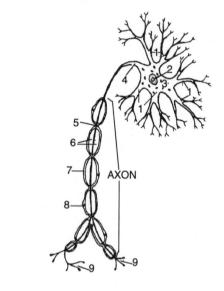

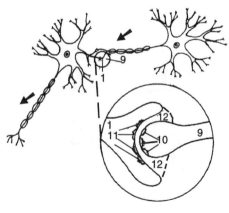

and white matter, is below par and below normal. Hence, the body is in a good deal worse condition than we have had." 5707-1 (my emphasis)

NERVES AS WE KNOW THEM

Basically, we have two primary nervous systems. One functions in response to *deliberate* action, such as walking, talking, and eating. It is called the central nervous system or cerebrospinal system. The other functions *automatically*, without thought or action on our part, such as breathing, digesting food, sleeping, and circulating the blood. It is called the autonomic nervous system, consisting of the sympathetic and parasympathetic systems. Under healthy conditions, these two systems work well together. For example, if you deliberately decide to go for a walk, you engage parts of the central nervous system (such as, those controlling muscle and bone); as you use them the autonomic system begins to make "sympathetic" adjustments in your body to aid in your walk, such as automatically increasing the supply of oxygen to the body, releasing some sugars from the liver to give you the needed energy, and so on. If you deliberately decide to go to sleep, the central system gets you there and the autonomic system makes sympathetic adjustments to put your body in a deep rest state.

As with blood, nerves are actually cells. They are specialized cells that link together in tiny branchlike structures. These structures have two parts: message receivers and message senders. A nerve cell is a combination of chemical and electrical power. When a nerve cell is at rest, it contains negatively charged potassium ions, and the fluid outside contains positively charged sodium ions. That is, of course, if the body has the proper potassium and sodium balance. In less than 1,000th of a second, this nerve cell can fire off a burst of chemicals that cause the positive-negative electrical charges to change. As this positive-negative flip-flop process moves through the branchlike structure, it ultimately causes a jump to the next branch, causing it to fire a burst that changes the negative-positive condition, and the message continues to move until it reaches the central coordinator of the entire body, the brain.

THE BRAIN

An adult brain weighs about three pounds. It is made up of gray matter and white matter. The gray matter consists of nerve-cell bodies. White matter consists of the connecting-communicating links among all these nerve cells (axons, dendrites, and glia). The brain is divided into three parts: the forebrain, midbrain, and hindbrain.

The forebrain is the deeply grooved portion that most of us know from pictures. Actually, this deeply grooved portion, called the cerebral cortex, is only about a ¼ inch thick. If we flattened out the cerebral cortex, it would be 2½ feet long and composed of 10 billion cells! It is divided into four lobes. The frontal lobes are the area where complex thoughts, decisions, and judgments concerning right and wrong are processed, just behind the forehead. (For us mystics, the third-eye area.) The frontal lobes also send messages to tell the body's muscles when and how to move. Behind the frontal lobes are the parietal lobes, where some information from the senses is processed. Below the parietal lobes lie the temporal lobes, where the speech center is located. It is where the brain makes sense of spoken and written language. Behind all of this lies the occipital lobes, where information from the eyes is processed. Below the cerebral cortex covering and its four lobes are the two great hemispheres of the brain (simply called, the right and left).

The two hemispheres are linked together by a ribbon of connecting fibers called the corpus callosum. In animals the two hemispheres function similarly. But in humans these hemispheres specialize their functions. This specialization is in a crossover manner, the left hemisphere controlling the right side of the body, the right hemisphere the left side. But they also divide the labor further. Studies have shown that the left half of the brain is more linear in its processing and the right half more holistic. The left hemisphere for most people handles the function of language and language-related capabilities, such as speech. Besides being verbal, the left half is analytical, sequential, symbolic, linear, and objective. The right half is very fast in its perceptions, and perceives things in a spatial, all-encompassing manner, as though it is seeing everything at once. It is imaginative, metaphorical, dreamlike, intuitive, spontaneous, relational, not sensitive to time, and subjective. However, the right brain is incapable of verbalizing what it is perceiving; for this it needs the left half. Messages go back and forth between these two hemispheres, creating a view and understanding of what's going on that is amazing. Though they use the same sensory system, they handle the information in different ways, thus yielding a bigger and better picture of what's really happening. However, the right half can use the "mind's eye" to perceive something beyond what's coming in through the senses. Furthermore, the hemispheres can be trained and developed, improving their unique skills and cooperative operation! For one example of this, see the great little book, *Drawing on the Right Side of the Brain* by Betty Edwards.

The midbrain contains the hypothalamus, pituitary gland, and pineal body, among other things. Here are the master hormonal controllers of the body, where growth, temperature, water balance, sexual behavior, and so on are regulated. In this area of the brain is also where dopamine is produced, the substance that regulates muscle rigidity and prevents muscles from trembling. We might consider this area of the brain as the chemical center, or hormonal center.

Below the midbrain is the hindbrain, which is in three parts: medulla oblongata (a bulb at the spinal cord's top), the cerebellum (shaped like two linked hemispheres), and the pons (a ridgelike bridge connecting the two spheres of the cerebellum). The hindbrain is the center of the control of the body's most basic functions, such as regulating the heartbeat, breathing, blood pressure, and other vital functions.

In four hollow spaces within the brain (ventricles) a very special liquid (cerebrospinal fluid) moistens and cushions the brain, and chemically connects it to the spinal column.

Messages between the brain and other parts of the head move along a network of 12 pairs of main nerves called cranial nerves, whose roots are directly within the brain. The 12 pairs of cranial nerves are responsible for eye movement, sensation in the face, jaws and teeth, facial expressions and movements, hearing and balance, taste, swallowing, and moving the tongue. However, the 10th pair of these nerves (the vagus nerve) actually descends down into the body, controlling the voice box (larynx), heart, lung, stomach functions, among other things. (For us mystics, these 12 paired nerves are the twenty-four elders in the biblical book of The Revelation, which Cayce encouraged us to spiritualize. More on this in the meditation section.)

THE BRAIN

1. Cerebral cortex
2. Cerebellum
3. Pons
4. Medulla oblongata
5. Spinal cord
6. Midbrain
7. Protective
   membranes

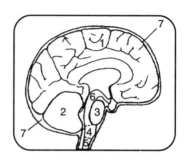

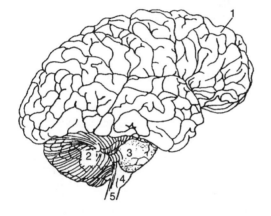

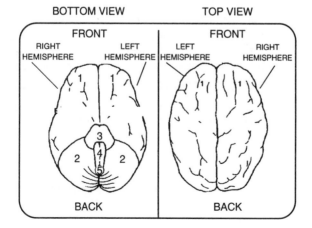

BOTTOM VIEW   TOP VIEW

FRONT   FRONT

RIGHT HEMISPHERE LEFT HEMISPHERE LEFT HEMISPHERE RIGHT HEMISPHERE

BACK   BACK

43

THE SPINAL CORD

The brain communicates with the rest of the body through 31 pairs of nerves branching off of the spinal cord. This is the main conduit for brain-body communication. The spinal cord is about 18 inches long, running from the base of the brain down the back, inside the bones of the spinal column. Like the brain, it is bathed in the special cerebrospinal fluid. Like the brain, it contains both gray and white matter. Once the main spinal cord nerves branch off, they continue to branch again and again in a network that reaches every area of the body, and keeping the whole body in constant communication with the brain. That is, if everything is flowing freely and in proper balance.

THE SYMPATHETIC NERVOUS SYSTEM

The branching network I've just described is the cerebrospinal system, or central nervous system. As we know, there is another, deeper nervous system that is critical to our health and rejuvenation. Cayce always called it the sympathetic system, but it is normally called the autonomic system. This system controls and coordinates breathing, digesting, maintaining blood pressure, regulating heartbeat, and many other things. This system is also in contact with the glands and organs of the body. The amazing thing about this system is that it can be stimulated by emotions, and cause the body to react physically to these emotions, by becoming fearful, angry or, preferably, calm. When a person is angry, tense, emotional, or startled, the brain automatically begins sending messages to the sympathetic portion of this nervous system. These messages tell the body to cope with these unpleasant circumstances. This may cause the adrenal glands to drop one of their powerful hormones (adrenaline or epinephrine) which would raise the heart rate and blood pressure, shunt extra blood to the limbs, increase sweating, and prepare the body to meet the emergency the brain perceives. On the other hand, if the brain perceives no danger, the body is well fed, and life in general is safe and pleasant, it sends a signal that causes the parasympathetic system to distribute relaxing messages (i.e., acetylcholine) throughout the glands and organs. The heart rate slows, the blood vessels relax, peace spreads throughout the system.

This leads us to the powerful glands, and their

SPINAL CORD

C1-C8. Cervical nerves
T1-T12. Thoracic nerves (dorsal)
L1-L5. Lumbar nerves
S1-S5. Sacral nerves

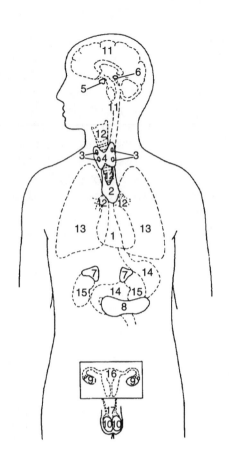

THE ENDOCRINE SYSTEM

1. Heart
2. Thymus gland
3. Parathyroid gland
4. Thyroid gland
5. Pituitary gland
6. Pineal gland
7. Adrenal gland
8. Pancreas
9. Ovaries (female)
10. Testes (male)
11. Brain and spinal cord
12. Trachea and bronchus
13. Lungs
14. Stomach
15. Kidneys
16. Uterus and fallopian tubes (female)
17. Scrotum (male)
Note: The cells of Leydig are found in the sexual glands and the adrenal glands.

role in health and rejuvenation.

THE GLANDS

The glands are the master messengers of the body. They use chemical forces to affect changes throughout the system. Here are two of Cayce's key comments on the glands:

> "All the elements for revivifying, or for producing reproduction of functioning of organs, activities, nerve forces, are produced by glands. Hence, the condition has been and is dependent upon the resuscitating of the influences [of the glands]. Hence the stimulation necessary along the cerebrospinal system, and the adjustments, as to allow the perfect flow of activity through the nerve impulses of ganglia activity. And, as the system is builded for better general health in assimilation, in distribution, it will aid the glands in producing or performing their necessary functions." 360-4

> "There must be those attentions to the body that will change the chemical reactions in which the glandular system takes from the body-forces, or the diet in the assimilation, to create the supplying elements for re-suscitating and revivifying of the affected areas." 3543-1

GLANDS AS WE KNOW THEM TODAY

There are two types of glands, exocrine and endocrine. The exocrine glands have ducts that direct their products to specific locations. Sweat glands, salivary glands, and the liver are examples. The ductless endocrine glands produce substances that go directly into the blood system, reaching the entire body within a minute or less. The endocrine gland system consist of the testes/ovaries, cells of Leydig, adrenals, pancreas, thymus, thyroid and parathyroid, pineal body, and the master gland, the pituitary.

For Edgar Cayce, the endocrine glands represented a major spiritual presence in the physical organism. He stated that the subconscious mind and the soul make their presence in the physical body through the autonomic nervous system, particularly through the sympathetic system. He went on to imply that the spiritual forces were in the body through the powerful endocrine glandular system. These ideas are difficult to accept given our modern focus on physical realities, with little or no awareness of subtle, nonphysical soul and spirit forces, especially within the physical organism. If we can't touch it, see it, or dissect it, then it doesn't exist. Some researchers accept that an unseen force can make its presence known through its effects, but few are looking for the effects of soul and spirit in the human. Yet, Cayce clearly says that they are there, and specifically identifies the autonomic nervous system and the endocrine glandular system as their place of influence. More on this in the section on meditation.

HORMONES

Hormones are the product of the endocrine system. This word comes from the Greek word *horman*, which means to "stir up." These powerful messages regulate the activity of the vital organs and functions of the body, from sex to sleep, from fight to flight, from growth to no growth, and much more.

In the Middle Ages, "humors" were believed to cause various dispositions in a person's mood or attitude and emotions. These humors were identified with four bodily fluids: blood, phlegm, bile, and choler. A sanguine person (cheerful, hopeful) was often ruddy in complexion; therefore, blood was believed to have contributed to this disposition. A phlegmatic person (slow, unemotional, apathetic) was often found to have an excess of mucus; therefore, phlegm was believed to have contributed to this disposition. A bilious person (ill-humored, irritable, unhappy) was considered to have an excess of gall or bile (yellowish-brown or green substance) secreted from the liver and stored in the gall bladder. Normally, it is discharged in the duodenum and aids in digestion. A person who had too much bile often looked a little green and unhappy. A choleric person (angry, irate, irascible, or easily angered) was considered to have too much choler (yellow bile) in his or her system. This type of person often looked a little yellow, jaundiced, and bad tempered.

A whole "science" of health and wellness was built around the lack or excess of these humors in the body.

The humors have now given way to the hormones. Like the humors' concept of lack and excess, hormonal balance within a body is critical to the disposition of that body and its occupant. Starting well before birth and continuing on through life, hormones affect the condition and disposition of the body.

The hormone insulin, from little islet cells in the pancreas gland, are critical to digestion. Estrogen, progesterone, and testosterone are hormones, produced in the ovaries and testes, which determine the sexual characteristics (such as hairy or smooth skin) and sexual changes (such as puberty and menopause). Androgens increase muscular strength. There is even a sexual difference in brain anatomy due to the presence or absence of testosterone during stages of development in the brain. The most famous hormone is adrenaline, produced by none other than the adrenal glands (located on top of our kidneys). This is the fight-or-flight hormone. But the adrenals produce many other hormones, some contributing to the sexual nature, some to the strength, some to prevent the loss of sodium in the urine (remember, the nerves need positive sodium ions to communicate). The thyroid gland produces hormones that regulate the growth process. In countries where iodine in lacking in the diet, we find many enlarged thyroids, called goiters. The thyroid needs sufficient iodine to manufacture its chief hormone, thyroxine. To show how closely the glands monitor one another, the hypothalamus and pituitary keep close watch over the amount of thyroxine in the blood system. When it drops below acceptable levels, the pituitary secretes a thyroid-stimulating hormone (TSH) to kick it into gear. Thyroxine has a direct influence upon heart rate and metabolism. The thyroid also produces other important hormones, such as calcitonin which regulates the amount of calcium in the system. The master endocrine gland, the pituitary, can secrete hormones that actually regulate other hormones, as well as glands.

When it comes to repair and renewal of the body, we must take into consideration the glands and their powerful hormones. Getting them functioning well will contribute to the rejuvenation process.

BLOOD, NERVES, AND HORMONES

Not surprisingly, the endocrine system works in cooperation with the blood and nervous systems. The blood system is the main conduit of endocrine messages. The nervous system and the endocrine system work in very similar ways. For the most part the nervous system regulates the body through electrical rather than chemical forces. But certain portions of the nervous system actually produce chemical messengers called neurohormones. The endocrine system mostly regulates the body through chemical rather than electrical forces. But certain portions of the endocrine system directly influence electrical messages in the body.

The most important relationship among the blood, nervous, and endocrine systems is *feedback*. Each of these systems gives and receives feedback from and to one another, which helps each to determine what is needed to create or maintain an overall healthy condition.

RADIAL APPLIANCE
& WET CELL BATTERY

Cayce said that each of these devices is only a supplement to good thoughts, attitudes, emotions, diet, exercise, massage, hydrotherapy and spinal adjustments. As we have seen, the Cayce approach is a holistic approach, combining and coordinating body, mind and soul. A physical activity should be combined and coordinated with a good mental attitude and a soulful, spiritual attunement. Nevertheless, there are times when we need some help getting things right. These devices were designed to do just that.

THE RADIAL APPLIANCE

The Radial Appliance is often referred to in the Cayce material as the "radio-active device." (As I explained earlier, Cayce meant this term in reference to a radio's activity, not nuclear energy's radioactivity.) It was the most often recommended device in the Cayce material. It is not a battery and therefore does not produce any voltage, but relies on the voltage produced by the skin of the body. This may explain why Cayce said that this device should only be used by one person, never shared. Somehow, the skin's voltage interacts in such a way with the device that it aids in balancing the electrical patterns of the body.

This appliance is a small canister in which bars of

high-grade 60-carbon steel are nested in a bed of charcoal and separated by strips of glass. Electrical connectors are attached to these bars and then the wires go to the body. It is first placed in sunlight to, according to Cayce, "clarify" or "purify" the device, and then, when ready to be used, it is put in a small pail of ice and water, which causes the device to activate. The disks at the end of the wires are attached to wrists and ankles in a four-step rotation (complete instructions come with each device). Generally, Cayce suggested it be used for a period of six weeks, and then stopped for two weeks in order to allow the body to try to maintain the energy pattern that the device has helped initiate. During this two-week rest period, Cayce again suggested the Radial Appliance be placed out in the sun for a few hours to clarify it.

Cayce recommended the Radial Appliance as an aid to improving sleep patterns, dream consciousness, meditation consciousness, various bio-electrical imbalances, fears, anxieties, low energy, moodiness, and general well-being. If the body were also suffering some ailment, then he would recommend adding a solution jar to the device, which would introduce the electrical forces of one of four solutions that he recommended: gold, silver, camphor, or iodine, depending upon what the ailment was.

THE WET CELL BATTERY

The Wet Cell Battery was recommended as an aid in helping with more serious illnesses. The Wet Cell is a chemical battery and therefore it does generate a voltage. Interestingly, the Wet Cell's voltage is almost identical to the skin's voltage. We are talking about a very, very small voltage, in the realm of 25,000th of a volt. Where the Radial Appliance works as a result of the skin's own voltage, the Wet Cell actually introduces a voltage into the body. In almost all cases, the Wet Cell is used in conjunction with a solution jar and one of the four solutions mentioned above.

There are actually two types of Wet Cells—a normal-charged charcoal cell and a "heavy-charged" iodine version.

The normal-charged charcoal Wet Cell was the most commonly recommended. It is a large container in which chemicals are mixed with distilled water to create the chemical battery. The black electrical wire goes to a solution jar with one of the four solutions, and then onto a specific spot near the body's umbilicus (navel). The red lead wire goes to various spots along the spinal column. Complete instructions come with each device.

The heavy-charged iodine Wet Cell was recommended as an aid for the more serious illnesses, such as multiple sclerosis (case numbers: 5073-1, 5108-1, 5238-1, 5324-1, 5403-1), arthritis, including rheumatoid (5129-1, 5120-1, 5150-1, 5169-1), impaired locomotion (5179-1), polio aftereffects (5182-1), muscular atrophy (5193-1), cerebral palsy (5209-1), paralysis injuries (5208-1), Parkinson's disease (3468-3), asthenia (5289-1), diabetes (5341-1), goiter (5173-1), glands (5269-1), blepharitis (5301-1).

The heavy-charged cell has a chemical charge similar to the normal Wet Cell, but with larger portions and no charcoal. In this chemical bath a 7% solution of iodine is suspended, and then the whole unit is given an added charge from a 6-volt battery charger. Solution jars and solutions are also involved, usually with gold chloride in the solution jar. Complete instructions come with each device.

The above material could not have been put together without the benefit of the wonderful research conducted by David McMillin and Douglas Richards, Ph.D., and presented in their book: *The*

Radial Appliance and Wet Cell Battery. (For information about this book or the appliances, please contact A.R.E. Member Services at 1-800-333-4499, or write to P.O. Box 595, Virginia Beach, VA 23451-0595.)

Chapter 3

Diet

Edgar Cayce used foods as medicines. He would change the chemistry of the body by changing the foods ingested by the body. He had an amazing insight into the effects of various foods upon the body, including the effect on the acid-alkaline balance. And, when one part of the digestive system wasn't functioning, he immediately called for adjustments to re-engage that part into the overall digestive process. In one discourse, he stated that if there was proper digestion, assimilation, and waste elimination, then the body could go on forever—that is, if the mind could keep interested in going on.

The following discourses are representative of Cayce's concepts, guidelines, and specific instructions about diet, various foods, and preparation methods.

"We would be mindful of the diet, that it consists principally of those of seafoods; of much that grows ABOVE the ground, as of the spinach, lettuce, and such GREEN vegetables. Any of the salads that carry large quantities of iron. Now this, apparently, would be the creat-

ing of blood, but blood of a character is needed."
5667-1

"Do use a good deal of seafood, a great deal of leafy vegetables, and the character of foods that are body and blood building; as celery, lettuce, radish, carrots, beets, beet tops, watercress—all of these should be taken quite often; not every day, to become tiresome for the body, but these will be found to be most helpful." 3043-1

"At present the diet would be those of the nature carrying the greater rebuilding forces in bloodstream and in nerve tissue. Much then of green vegetable forces, and fish, that are necessary for the body's development. Little of those of starchy or of the heavy forces." 3837-1

"There needs to be the care of the diet, for those conditions as necessary for the BUILD-ING of blood, of strength, of vitality, of muscle; and the body with this kind of food—not the highly seasoned, but that of the nutritious nature: Fish, fowl, and much vegetable; celery, lettuce, and the vegetables green as much as possible. Cornbread (not white bread), whole wheat bread." 5618-5

"In tomatoes there is found the three NEC-ESSARY vitamins for growth and for DEVEL-OPMENT. The same is seen in carrots—save these are not BALANCED in the same ratio as in tomatoes—but THESE may be given in the raw state. With tomatoes, choose the well ripe (vine ripened). Another WELL balanced food with THIS . . . is spinach, well cooked, with no oil or grease save butter. This will furnish another vitamin, an iron that is excellent for the blood. Well too that those of the glutens be used, which will be found by rolling wheat, raw wheat, see? and this cooked as a gruel—a little salt and little butter, and a very SMALL quantity of sugar." 5520-2

"In the matter of diet—these should be nerve and blood building, but do not force self to eat that as is not desirous of being eaten! Do not over STIMULATE the system with those of any character of foods that supply overabundance of sugars, or overabundance of alcoholic forces, as when there are those of fruits and fruit juices taken, do not take those that produce fermentations within the system; for these unbalance the ASSIMILATING forces of the system, as does overacidity or too highly seasoned foods." 5423-1

"The activity of the olive oil [as a massage oil] is as FOOD that may be absorbed by the lymph and emunctories of the system, provided the pores and the exterior portions of the body have been relaxed or opened before this is massaged into the system. The activity of those properties as go WITH same, the myrrh and those of sassafras oil, these add to the STRENGTH of the muscular tissue, of the sinew along the system, as to carry—the one stimulating the muscular forces, the other carrying to the cartilaginous forces, and to every nerve fiber itself, that of strength and activity. The Gold in its activity, with the Soda, is to ENLIVEN the glands INTERNALLY with the SECRETIONS of the system, as to furnish the proper stimuli to the replenishing and rebuilding of the system.

"Q: Are the sores on face caused from sugar in the blood?

57

"A: Rather from the lack of GLUTEN [from wheat] in the blood, that KEEPS the eliminating system in coordination. With the strengthening of the vitality of the nerve ends of the nervous system, with the stimuli to the glands of the body in every direction, we will find these conditions will disappear—but the WARNINGS, as given, do NOT take properties that make for too much sugars or too much of the stimuli in that of ACIDITY in the system." 5423-1

"Fruits, vegetables are better, but not much of meats. One meal each day, whether morning, evening or in the noon, one whole meal should consist of RAW vegetables. Combine these of all the leafy and all those vegetables that may be combined in a salad. Lettuce, celery, carrots, beans, spinach, onions, cabbage, and or all of these. Such a salad may be changed occasionally to a whole FRUIT meal; as apples, oranges, peaches, lemons, pears—don't put in any bananas! All of these may be combined and used instead of the meal of vegetables. Meats if they are taken at all should never be fried; in fact, NO FRIED FOODS AT ALL!" 1204-2

Much of what he says fits with what we've come to know today. The human body does better with fruits and vegetables, than with too much meat and fats. Deep fried foods are very hard to digest. Mixing certain foods makes digestion difficult. However, one of his key examples is something our society promotes: orange juice and milk at the same meal. My own common sense tells me these two are incompatible. But they are promoted as parts of a complete breakfast.

VITAMINS

Occasionally, Cayce would recommend taking vitamin supplements, but his more common approach was to add foods to the diet that were rich in whatever vitamin was needed.

"Do add more strengthening foods to the body-forces in the diets which carry E vitamins as well as A and B or the B-complex or B-combinations, niacin and iron. For we must enrich the blood from the deteriorations that are beginning to indicate how a form of anemia is affecting the resistances of the body.

"Do follow the diets in foods which are rich in necessary minerals for replenishing blood supply. The E vitamin, the wheat germ with the cereals or wheat germ oil taken in capsule at least once a week or twice during the week. Best that it be varied, one week once-a-week, next week twice-a-week, next week three times, but have regular periods for it. The B-1 should be rich in the foods which are taken. We would find this from all foods which are yellow in color, not as greens that would turn yellow, but as the yellow variety of squash, carrots, wax beans, peaches, all of these are well. Though, there are other foods, to be sure, as liver, beef juices, fish, all of these are well to be portions of the diet." 5319-1

In some of Cayce's discourses he actually stated that the use of vitamin supplements was a waste, until the system was corrected to be able to assimilate them, as in this next discourse:

"The continual taking of such [B-complex vitamins] will do very little good, unless the system is so adjusted that these may be assimilated so that the strength and vitality may go into the system through glandular activity and be distributed through blood and nerve supply. When the corrections are made [adjustments to spine and reduction of toxins in system] these supplementary vitamins may be taken (not in the beginning) and assimilated by the body so as to gain strength." 5017-1

IONIZING FOODS

"Alternate between those foods that carry a large percentage of iron and those that carry assimilated ionized forces as with iodine. Or let most of the foods now be with fish, shell fish or the like." 1225-3

"Q: Would you recommend any specific diet?
"A: The fresh vegetables, raw vegetables, are preferable to meats; for the body needs the balancing throughout the system of the centralizing system being kept ionized as related to the eliminations of the body." 865-1

"Too much calcium in the system, too much potash, and not sufficient amount of iodine as related to the ironizing and oxidization as take place in the system." 51-1

Cayce's reference to too much calcium and too much potash is very interesting. Both of these are inorganic minerals (neither animal nor vegetable) in structure. They both form as an ash when animal or plant materials are burned. When burned, the organic portions of animals and plants are gone, easily assimilated into the biosphere, but an ash remains. Apparently, Cayce is equating the outer burning of animals and plants with the inner burning of them in our digestive processes. Potash is a term associated with potassium, particularly certain types of potassium. Although it is an important mineral for the body, too much or too little potassium is known to result in cardiac arrhythmias. Sources of potassium are bananas, oranges, apricots, avocados, potatoes, bran, peanuts, and dried peas and beans. Sources of calcium are milk, cheese, and seafoods (mussels, oysters, salmon, shrimp, etc.). Of course, these same seafoods also provide iodine. Perhaps case #51 was ingesting too much of the milk and dairy sources of calcium without getting enough iodine.

"Change the diet, keeping the oils—not only the olive oil, but those of the cod-liver oil, to replenish the blood supply. IRONIZING the whole system, as it were." 5554-2

CARBON FOOD

"It is better for the body to eat oftener instead of in large quantities. He should not eat so much of a starch, but more of a property that will produce carbon to the body, so that it will not burn itself out." 5707-1

"[We need] plenty of carbon, oxygen for the system, so the body can be re-ironized. Plenty of those food values that carry much of iron and iodine, reducing potashes in the system, as to relieve nerve tension." 5554-2

"A diet of a nature of carbons to the system to rebuild or rejuvenate the blood forces. The iron and calcium into the system will produce more of a system to call fuel for the system." 4801-1

"Occasionally, the body has too much carbon, as in this case:

"Keep the diet in that way and manner that will produce at all times the easy digestion. Not too much of fuels or carbons, or carbohydrates, but more of the protein and vegetable forces that give the tissue in the white blood and lymphatic forces." 4988-2

As I pointed out earlier, Cayce seems to be using the term "carbon" in a manner similar to how we use "carbohydrate." However, in 5707-1, he does seem to be differentiating a true carbon food from a starchy food. Carbohydrates [literally a combination of the words "carbon" and "water"] are formed from carbon, hydrogen, and oxygen through a complex process in which plants with green leaves transform energy from the sun. The plant uses some of the carbohydrate for its own needs; the rest is stored in various parts—seeds, leaves, stalks, roots, tubers, and so on. This stored carbohydrate can easily be broken down, digested, and assimilated into our systems, yielding its rich values to our bodies. Carbohydrates are in whole-grain bread, pasta, and cereal; and fruits, berries, some vegetables, maple sap, honey, sugars (beet, cane, etc.), and milk. In fact, there is a vast array of foods that contain carbohydrates. It appears that Cayce would prefer we use carbohydrates that do not contain starch, but yield a pure carbon influence when digested. When we study his recommended diet, it does not contain pastas and processed breads. It does contain whole-grain cereals, fruits, and vegetables. These would appear to be the better sources of carbon.

ACID & ALKALINE BALANCE

"In the matter of the diets: Here we need body-building foods, but those that tend to be more alkaline-producing than acid—for the natural inclinations of disturbed conditions in a body are to produce acidity through the bloodstream. Hence, we need to REVIVIFY same by the use of much of those that produce more of the enzymes, more of the hormones for the blood supply; yet not overburdening the body with those unless the balance in the vitamin forces is carried." 1302-1

"Those that are blood and nerve building, and may be changed to any of the characters of foods that are ALKALINE REACTING! Eggs may be taken at this time, provided the YOLK only is prepared, either in the form of hard and WELL MASHED afterward, mixed with any of the oils—olive oil, also those of cod-liver oil, should be part of the diet." 5520-2

"Do set up the alkalinizing of body and the eliminations of poisons." 5319-1

"As to the diet, keep more of the alkalines. No heavy foods that EVER are fried. And let one meal each day be of only raw green vegetables; not green in color necessarily, but in their very nature—those that carry all the vitamins necessary in creating the effluvia within the blood and nerve supply that is revivifying in its very nature." 743-1

Sometimes the body can become too alkaline, as in this comment:

"There has become an excess of alkalinity, and thus, through the digestive system, there is a lack of sufficient of the acids to produce proper digestions in the system." 3481-3

This comment brings us to the digestive system. I have found that it helps to know our bodies and how they function. Now that we know more about the blood, nervous, and glandular systems, it would help us if we understood how our bodies digest food. You might recall Cayce's comments in case 681-2 where he states that a balance between assimilation and elimination will keep a body going forever! Let's take a moment to understand how we assimilate and eliminate properly.

THE DIGESTIVE SYSTEM

Good digestion begins with food selection. Food to our bodies comes in three basic forms: carbohydrates (sugars and starches), proteins, and fats.

Carbohydrates are the main source of food energy for people all over the world. In some countries carbohydrates make up 80 to 90 percent of the diet—in Asia this would be from rice, in Europe it would be from bread, in Ireland and England it would be from potatoes. In the U.S.A. about 40 to 50 percent of our diet is carbohydrates.

There are two main categories of carbohydrates: sugars and starches. Sugars can be converted into starches for long-term storage. Plants store much of this in their seeds and roots, but animals (of which we are one) store much of this in their livers. Plants use carbohydrates for structural building, but animals use protein for this. Animals use carbohydrates and fats for energy food.

When oxygen from the air is combined with various foods, the result is oxidation or burning. The energy that is released is measured in calories. Caloric energy is used to do work, from big work to simply supplying the chemical reactions for the body's normal functioning. A gram of carbohydrate will put out about 4 calories of energy, whereas a gram of fat will put out 9 calories.

The best carbohydrate foods are those that contain other nutrients. Potatoes, rice, corn, and whole-grain bread also supply protein, vitamins, and minerals along with their complex carbohydrates. However, table sugar, honey, syrup (even corn syrup), and soda pops are almost pure carbohydrates. This is why they are called "empty calories." They provide nothing more to the body than calories. The good carbohydrates come from fruits, vegetables, whole grains, and nuts. But one has to watch out for added sweeteners. In most cereals today they add hundreds of empty calories in the form of brown sugar, corn sweetener, corn syrup, dextrose, fructose, fruit juice concentrate, glucose, honey, the famous "high fructose corn syrup," lactose, maltose, maple syrup, molasses, raw sugar, sucrose, sugar, syrup, and a host of artificial sweeteners, such as: saccharin, aspartame, sorbitol, and mannitol.

For most carbohydrates, Cayce liked to have them picked and eaten after they have ripened, not before (especially fruits and vegetables, most notably tomatoes). He also said, "Vegetables, unlike people, are better the fresher they are." He liked the grains cooked well with plenty of water, even into a gruel. This would release most all of the gluten from the cells of the grain, making it readily digestible. He often recommended cooking methods that would retain vitamins and minerals which would normally be lost into the cooking water. One was the use of patapar paper. On this cooking topic, he was most upset about the growing use of aluminum in cooking pans. He stated that foods cooked in aluminum are changed in a way that makes them unhealthy.

As you may have already noticed, carbohydrates provide the bulk of our necessary dietary fiber; that is, if we eat the whole thing. Whole grains have their fibrous bran, and unpeeled fruits still have their fiber. For example, a whole apple has 3.6 grams of fiber, but applesauce has only 0.2 grams. White rice and white bread have little to none of their original bran fiber present.

Proteins are the main growth, repair, and replacement food for animals (which includes us). Meat, fish, eggs, cheese, beans, dried peas and similar vegetables, and some grains are the main sources for protein. Cayce always recommended less red meats, and more fish, fowl, or lamb. Of course, vegetables were high on his list of good food.

Fats are rich in energy and are needed in the body in small amounts. The main sources of fats are milk, butter, cheese, meats, olives, peanuts, sunflower seeds, and soy beans. Most dieticians believe that plant fats are better for us than animal fats, as does Cayce. But too much of any fat is bad for us and our hearts.

Vitamins come from fresh vegetables, citrus fruits, other fruits, and berries. Vitamins are critical for growth, repair, and vital functions. For example, vitamin A is needed for growth, resistance to infection, and maintaining healthy skin and eyes, while vitamin K is essential for blood clotting. Vitamins A, K, D, and E are fat soluble and can therefore be stored in the liver. But B and C vitamins are water soluble and because of the way the kidneys filter water, they cannot be stored in the body and must therefore be provided in the diet regularly.

Minerals are critical for nerve communication (sodium and potassium), releasing energy from foods (phosphorus), building bones and teeth (calcium), and many other bodily functions. Minerals come from whole grains, legumes (beans, lentils), and some fruits and vegetables.

Digestion begins as soon as the eye or nose gets excited by the sight or smell of food. The mouth begins to salivate, and saliva is the first important step to thorough digestion and assimilation. Cayce often encouraged people to produce more saliva, chew their food more thoroughly, and mix saliva with their foods and even their drinks. Food and drink move down the esophagus and into the stomach, where they are combined with mucus, hydrochloric acid, and powerful enzymes. The acid in the stomach softens food and destroys any germs in the food. The powerful enzyme pepsin begins to break down proteins and prepares them for digestion. In the stomach food is changed into a soupy substance called chyme. Small amounts of chyme are rhythmically squirted through a ring-like muscle (pyloric sphincter) into the next section of the digestive system: the duodenum (pronounced, du-od-dennum). Here the highly acidic chyme is neutralized by alkali. This also stops the action of the enzyme pepsin, which only works in an acid environment. Now alkaline enzymes take over. Two small tubes connect the pancreas and the gall bladder to the duodenum. The gall bladder secretes the bile made by the liver into the duodenum. Bile emulsifies blobs of fat in the chyme. The pancreas secretes more enzymes, some of which digest the emulsified fats, some continue to break down proteins, some work on carbohydrates. The pancreas also secretes the hormone insulin into the duodenum. As we know, insulin helps to control the amount of sugar in the bloodstream and the way cells use energy. Much digestion has now taken place, but little to no assimilation of the nutrients into the body. This occurs in the small intestine. Here the blood system and the lymph get into the action, and begin to carry some of the nutrients to the body. In the lining of the small intestine is a rich blood supply, which allows the blood to carry the nutrients off. By now the food has become molecules of amino acids (from proteins), sugars (carbohydrates), and triglycerides (from fat).

Triglycerides tend to pass through the lacteal ducts of the lymphatic system rather than the blood system. The blood vessels carry the amino acids and sugars to the liver—some for storage, some however go on throughout the body for immediate use.

Digestion ends with the small intestine and elimination begins with the large intestine or bowel (as in bowel movement). As the largely indigestible materials pass through the large intestine, water and mineral salts are absorbed through the intestinal lining into the body. As this occurs, the material in the intestine becomes less fluid and changes into the brownish, semi-solid feces or stools that will eventually be eliminated from the body. About ⅓ of the fecal matter is fiber, another third is dead bacteria, and the final third consists of unwanted mineral salts, mucus, bile contents, and rubbed-off bits of intestinal lining.

Remember the vagus nerve, the tenth of the twelve paired brain nerves? It controls the digestive process. This nerve controls everything from appetite to churning up the stomach, from speeding up the flow to slowing it down, from secreting the necessary hormones and digestive juices to decisions about storing or using the energy in the food.

Cayce often quoted the old saying, "After breakfast, work awhile; after lunch, rest awhile; after dinner, walk a mile." The rest allows the body to fully devote its attention to digestion and assimilation before working again. However, since few of us work in the evenings, it is best to walk off the dinner before retiring, when the digestive system slows down, leaving the meal a drag on the system.

THE DIGESTIVE SYSTEM

1. Teeth
2. Salivary glands
3. Tongue
4. Epiglottis
(keeps air and
food separate)
5. Esophagus
6. Trachea
7. Stomach

8. Spleen
9. Liver
10. Diaphragm
11. Gallbladder
12. Pancreas
13. Small intestine
14. Appendix
15. Large Intestine
16. Rectum

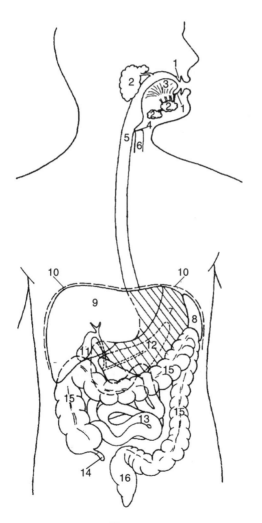

Chapter 4

EXERCISE AND REST

FRESH AIR WALKS

"
[Be in the] air, sand, and water. These are needed more for the body than any other condition—sunshine and shadows. The body needs to get CLOSE to nature, with nature's curers—as will be found in sand, sunshine, water, woods. Such natures as this, and we will find, in three to four weeks, with such care of self, such taking of sunshine baths, of sand baths, of walks in wood, of communing with nature, and of introspection of self and duty to self and that owed to mankind and to God, through the efforts of the individuals themselves, there will be brought strength, power, force, vitality. Do that." 5618-5

"We must have more oxygen, so that the lungs will throw off the carbon from the body. He should be more outdoors, and take more bodily exercise; have more employment of the mind, to get it off of self, or to do something that will relax the body, not enough of course to wear it out—then the body will rebuild." 5707-1

"Enliven the supplying of carbon and of the oxidized oxygen or ozone to the blood supply as reached through the lung forces, see?" 4790-1

"In the blood supply to the body we find this in the lungs proper does not receive the sufficient carbon to supply the system." 4550-1

SLEEP

"Sleep is the building time of the physical forces to give and partake of rejuvenal expressions." 5681-1

"Well that the irrigations of oil be occasionally used for the lower portion of the system, so that the colon may be cleansed properly, and that the STRAIN as has been induced by the lack of blood supply through this portion of the system may be increased. BUILD up the general system.

"The manipulations (osteopathic/chiropractic) as would be given in this condition would be for the strengthening of the whole nerve system, that the body may relax thoroughly when it rests—for the BUILDING properties for THIS body will be found in rest and sleep." 5520-2

Before moving on from the physical aspects of the body to a deeper look at meditation, I'd like to quote one of the most amazing comments by Cayce:

"It should be considered by all: There is no greater factory in the universe than a human body in its natural, normal reacting state. For there are those machines or glands within the body capable of producing, from the very air, water and food values taken into the body to reproduce ANY element AT ALL that is KNOWN in the material world!" 1800-21

Obviously we have the right equipment to do the job of rejuvenation. The body is an amazing "factory" when it is functioning in its natural and normal state. Our job is to get it there, and then maintain it—and to do so for a good purpose.

Chapter 5

MEDITATION—
A UNIQUE REJUVENATOR

As we saw earlier in this book, Edgar Cayce considered the practice of meditation to be a major aid to rejuvenation.

> "Being able to raise **within** the vibrations of individuals to that which is a resuscitating, a revivifying influence and force **through the deep meditation** (the attunement of self to the higher vibrations in Creative Forces), these are manifested in man through the promises that are coming from Creative Forces or Energy itself!" 993-4 (bold is author emphasis but Cayce's parenthetical comment)

For all of us who want to realize the benefits of meditation, let me outline some important ingredients in a successful meditation practice. For clarity, let's confine our study to techniques and theories in two methods of meditation, Magic Silence and Kundalini—each described in varying detail in the Cayce volumes.

Before we begin, we must be clear that meditation is an *altered* state of consciousness. It is not a method for getting our normal consciousness to feel better. As Cayce explains, "You don't have the meditation because . . . you want to feel better, but to attune self to the Infinite!" (1861-18) We must set our normal, everyday selves aside and allow our deeper, spiritual selves to awaken. This is perhaps the most fundamental and yet the most difficult requirement of meditation. But it can be done. The body, mind, and soul are interconnected in such a way that certain actions will automatically lead to "the magic silence" (137-3) and the awakening of our better selves.

THE TWO NERVOUS SYSTEMS

According to Cayce, our outer, everyday selves function mostly through the central nervous system of our bodies. As we have seen, this system includes portions of the brain, the spinal cord, the musculoskeletal system, and the five senses. We control this system with our conscious minds—choosing to walk, talk, smell, or touch whenever we care to. However, there is another system within our bodies that is under the control of our subconscious. This is the autonomic nervous system. It consists of the sympathetic/parasympathetic system, the organs and glands of the body, including the endocrine glands, which Cayce identifies with the spiritual centers, the chakras. The subconscious and its companion, the soul, are overseeing the temperature, chemistry, fuel needs, heartbeat, breathing, assimilation, digestion; and reacting to the needs and demands of the outer system.

ACTIONS THAT LEAD INWARD

What do these two nervous systems have to do with successful meditation? When we quiet the outer system and do something to stimulate the inner system, we are setting aside our outer selves and actually activating our souls. For example, let's sit down and stop using our musculoskeletal systems. Let's reduce our sense perception by closing down our five senses—close our eyes, stop touching, listening, smelling, and tasting. This quiets the outer system and the outer self. Now, let's take hold of some part of the inner system that the soul and subconscious have charge of, and let's *alter* it. The most popular part is the breath. The autonomic system, under the control of the subconscious mind and soul, is in charge of and directly connected to the breath. If we start changing the breath, we cause the soul and subconscious mind to become alert to these changes. This is an action that leads from our outer selves to our inner selves, and ultimately to an altered state of consciousness.

1. THE MAGIC SILENCE METHOD

Let's try this meditation method right now. Using a combination of an affirmation and a mantra, in coordination with a breathing pattern, we can enter into the magic silence. Let's use a modification of a line from Psalm 46 (often quoted by Cayce), "Be still and know God." In order to fully succeed with this affirmation/mantra, not only do we need the power of the words but we must take hold of the breath, and create a breathing pattern that arouses the soul. It works like this: "Be STILL [inhale slowly while feeling the word *Still* and exhale slowly] and know GOD [inhale slowly while feeling the word *God* and exhale slowly]." In between the phrases breathe in and out completely before going on to the next phrase. Keep the breath relaxed yet under your control.

If the feeling/breathing phase of this method is being experienced well, and no distractions are occurring, then do another breathing cycle before going onto the next phrase. If you are in the stillness or the Godness, remain in it as long as your conscious-ness holds there. If it moves, then bring it back by saying (in your mind) the next phrase. These silent periods between the phrases are the more impor-tant parts of this practice. The phrases gather and direct the consciousness but the spaces of silence are golden, or as Cayce calls them, "magical." So, as long as you are silent and still, stay there; don't feel a need to move on to the next phrase or repeat the phrases.

This method of combining an affirmation/man-tra with breathing will bring even the weakest medi-tator into a deep stillness and a heightened sense of Godness.

To move deeper, add three "OM's" (sounds like "om" in home) on the end of the last phrase: "Be STILL [feel and breathe], and know GOD [feel and breathe], OOOMMMM [feel and breathe] OOOMMMM [feel and breathe] OOOMMMM [feel and breathe]. This can be out loud in the beginning and then quiet in your mind as you go deeper. When chanting the OM incantation aloud, remember that true chant-ing is an *inner sounding,* not an outer singing. Keep the sound resonating within the cavities of your body. Beginning with the abdominal cavity, rising to the pulmonary cavity, and then on into the cra-nial cavity, let the sound carry you deeper.

I've taught this method to people who have never meditated before and had them in a deep silence for twenty minutes, coming out with that wonder-ful glaze in their eyes that results from an altered state. Their outer self is moved yet uncertain as to exactly what has happened. But they know they have just meditated well. I've also had people who had tried meditation for years with little success come out of one of these sessions with the biggest smiles on their faces—success at last!

THREE KEYS TO THIS METHOD

There are three keys to this method. First, the power of the words *still* and *God,* and their effect on us. Second, the connection between the breath and the soul—allowing us to arouse our souls by taking hold of the breathing pattern. Third, the spaces of silence between the words while breathing. These spaces grow longer and longer as one practices. Eventually, an hour's meditation is easy (and highly recommended by Cayce). According to him, and many other sources, the silence is in itself transforming. One need not "do" or "hear" anything when in meditation. Abide in the silence and it works its magic.

PHYSICAL CHANGES

Now we know from the research done in the '70s with TM (Transcendental Meditation) meditators and others, that the body goes through many changes during meditation. As researchers Wallace and Benson discovered, meditation causes measurable physical changes. "There is a reduction in oxygen consumption, carbon dioxide elimination, and the rate and volume of respiration; a slight increase in the acidity of the arterial blood; a marked decrease in the blood-lactate level; a slowing of the heartbeat; a considerable increase in skin resistance; and an electroencephalogram pattern of intensification of slow alpha waves with occasional theta-wave activity." (Wallace & Benson, 1973, p. 266)

Cayce's discourse 5752-3 expands on the wonderful changes: "Meditate . . . in the inner secrets of the consciousness, and the cells in the body become aware of the awakening of the life . . . " The cells of the body become aware? According to Cayce, every cell in the body has consciousness, and that consciousness may be raised or lowered. His discourse goes on, "In the mind, the cells of the mind become aware of the life in the spirit." The cells of the mind, life in the spirit? Interesting concepts, aren't they? "God is Spirit, and seeks same to worship Him" (John 4:23-24). Then, if raising the consciousness leads to awareness of "life in the spirit," it leads to life with God—the Great Spirit. The wonderful thing about this whole process is that we activate it by entering into the silence. Silence in itself is magical.

Now I would like us to look at another area of the total meditation picture. I would not recommend going on to this next practice until you have practiced the Magic Silence method with much success, and feel you are ready to go further with meditation. As with medicine so it is with meditation: one person's poison may be another's cure, and activities that may be harmful at one stage in life may be quite helpful at another. You have to judge what is best for you now, and continue to evaluate your readiness as you progress.

It may appear contradictory to say that silence is in itself transforming and then to describe another form of meditation in which inner activities are used to effect greater transformation, but such is the case with the Cayce method on meditation. The explanation for this is that the manifold nature of full enlightenment and transformation is such that contradiction and paradox are elements of any method. After all, we are dealing with celestial beings in terrestrial forms, spirits in flesh, godlings who are also human, eternal beings in temporary manifestations. Paradox and contradiction are bound to be a part of any process that attempts to resolve or integrate these.

Furthermore, as one progresses with their development, they naturally become more able to handle complexity and intricacy. They become more aware of and participate in the many aspects of the

Godhead, the Universal Consciousness, with all its diversity.

2. THE POWERFUL KUNDALINI METHOD

Like the Magic Silence method, this method will use words, breath, and spaces of silence, but in more powerful ways. Since there is more power involved, there are more warnings in the Cayce material about using this method without proper preparation and self-examination.

WARNINGS

Here's a typical warning from Cayce:

"Make haste SLOWLY! Prepare the body, prepare the mind, before ye attempt to loosen it in such measures or manners that it may be taken hold upon by those influences which constantly seek expressions of self rather than of a living, constructive influence of a CRUCI-FIED Savior. Then, crucify desire in self; that ye may be awakened to the real abilities of help-fulness that lie within thy grasp . . . without preparation, desires of EVERY nature may become so accentuated as to destroy." 2475-1

So, let's examine our purposes, search our hearts for our true passion. Is it cooperation and coordination with God, or are we still longing to gratify some lingering desires of our own self-interests?

The Taoist meditators of *The Secret of the Golden Flower* talk about the right method being like one wing of a bird, the other wing being the right heart. A wise seeker must remember, the bird cannot fly with one wing. All seekers must have the right method and the right heart.

THE IDEAL

The concept of the right heart leads us naturally to Cayce's teaching that an *ideal* should be raised as we seek to awaken the life force. What is our ideal? To whom or what do we look for examples of better behavior, better choices, better uses for our energies, better relating skills with others? What standard guides us in conceiving our better selves? Who is the author of our "Book of Life"? Is it the circumstances of life? Is it our self-interests? These are important questions from Cayce's perspective, questions that should be considered before going on with the powerful life forces that will be aroused in this method of meditation. As Cayce says, we can build a Frankenstein or a god using the same techniques. It all depends on the ideal held as the practice progresses.

JESUS CHRIST

The Cayce texts present Jesus Christ as not only the highest ideal but as a powerful force of protection for anyone seeking to loosen their life force to open the biospiritual seals and enter into the presence of the Divine. Christ is presented as an advocate for us before the Godhead. To call on this protection and guidance is to call on the greatest resource available. However, Cayce does not use Jesus Christ as a religion above other religions. His vision is too universal for that. Seekers from any religious faith can use the power of Christ in their meditative practice and still remain loyal to their religion. Here's an example of this perspective from Cayce:

"If there has been set the mark (mark meaning here the image that is raised by the individual in its imaginative and impulse force) such that it takes the form of the ideal the individual is holding as its standard to be raised to, ... then the individual (or the image) bears the mark of the Lamb, or the Christ, or the Holy One, or the Son, or any of the names we may have given to that which enables the individual to enter THROUGH IT into the very presence of that which is the creative force from within itself—see? Raising then in the inner self that image of the Christ, love of God-Consciousness, is making the body so cleansed as to be barred against all powers that would in any manner hinder." 281-13

Notice how Christ is explained as "love of God-Consciousness." Seekers from any religion may have love of God-Consciousness. Christ in this perspective is more universal than the religion that possesses the name. Notice also how "love of God-Consciousness" cleanses us of self-interests that may hinder or harm us.

However, there is much more to this excerpt than ecumenism and protection. Cayce is giving us a great insight into just how a meditator may be transported from a good meditative stillness into the very presence of the Creative Force, God—with all the rejuvenative ramifications of such an experience. If in our imaginative forces we can conceive or form the ideal (the standard) to which we seek to be raised, then we (as The Revelation states) bear the mark or the sign of that power (whatever name we give it) that enables us to enter through it into the very presence of God within us, the Creative Force within us. Despite the power of some of the other techniques in this form of meditation, imaging the ideal is seminal to transformation. Cayce points out the only limitation: "The entity is only limited to that it sets as its ideal." (1458-1) We are "gods in the making" if we can conceive ourselves to be such—in cooperation and coordination with the Great God.

THE KUNDALINI AND ETERNAL LIFE

The Cayce texts interweave Judeo-Christian-Islamic teachings found throughout the Old and New Testaments, but particularly in the book of The Revelation, with concepts and practices from ancient Hinduism and yoga. The fundamental concepts are these. The kundalini is metaphorically seen as the great serpent power fallen from its original place of honor. As Adam and Eve fell from grace in the Garden, so did the serpent. Yet, as Moses raised the serpent in the desert and Jesus raised it to life everlasting (John 3:14-15), so each of us must raise our serpent power to its rightful, original place of honor. Kundalini meditation is intended to do just that.

This kundalini or life force resides within the human body, which is the temple. Normally it is used in ways that dissipate the life force, eventually leading to aging and death of the body. Individuals are allowed to use their life force as they choose (at least within the parameters of their karma). Whether they dissipate it consciously or unconsciously makes no difference. When it's gone, it's gone. But it doesn't have to be this way. As Cayce puts it, " . . . if there will be gained that consciousness, there need not be ever the necessity of a physical organism aging . . . seeing this, feeling this, knowing this, ye will find that not only does the body become revivified, but by the creating in every atom of its being the knowledge of the activity of this Creative Force . . . spirit, mind, body [are] renewed." (1299-1)

The *élan vital* of the Western world or the "kundalini" of the Eastern world follows natural laws and can be made to flow in rejuvenative ways which enhance and extend the life. This is not only possible with kundalini meditation but it is a valuable goal to pursue. As we saw in an earlier excerpt that bears repeating here: "How is the way shown by the Master? What is the promise in Him? The last to be overcome is death. Death of what? The *soul* cannot die, for it is of God. The body may be revivified, rejuvenated. And it is to that end it may, the body, transcend the earth and its influence." (262-85) This meditation practice works directly with the forces of life.

THE SEVEN SPIRITUAL CENTERS OF THE BODY

In the Eastern teachings about meditation, there are seven chakras in the body that can be made to turn, like wheels, with a higher energy than is normally used. Cayce takes these Eastern chakras and connects them with the seven main endocrine gland centers in the human body. He does, however, change their order slightly, saying that the correct order was lost along the way, but was known during the origins of these mystical schools. Here is his list and order:

Pituitary	Highest Center	Forehead (Third Eye)
Pineal	6th Center	Crown of Head
Thyroid	5th Center	Throat
Thymus	4th Center	Chest (Heart Center)
Adrenals	3rd Center	Solar Plexus
Leydig Cells	2nd Center	Just Below the Navel
Gonads	1st Center	Ovaries or Testes

He says that the path of kundalini energy or the life force is in the shape of a raised king cobra or a shepherd's staff—running from the lower centers, up the spinal cord, into the base of the brain, over to the center of the brain, and then on to the forehead.

"The spirit and the soul is within its encasement, or its temple within the body of the individual—see? With the arousing, it rises along that which is known as the Appian Way, or the pineal center, to the base of the brain, that it may be disseminated to those centers that give activity to the whole of the mental and physical being. It rises then to the hidden eye in the center of the brain system [pituitary center], or is felt in the forefront of the head, or in the place just above the real face—or bridge of nose, see?" 281-13

PRAYER WORDS

Now let's look at the mechanics of this method. Assuming that our ideals, purposes, and hearts are in the right place, that we have crucified our selfish desires, conceived of our ideal, and drawn on the power and protection of the Christ, "love of God-Consciousness"—let's begin with prayer-words for the seven spiritual centers (or chakras). These words vary with different practices, but Cayce teaches that one reason the Master created the Lord's Prayer was for this purpose. And Cayce gives a slightly different version of the prayer, so let's try it. Cayce is also a proponent of the feminine aspect of the Godhead as well as the masculine, so let's also use this. As you say the prayer, feel the meaning of the words as your consciousness is directed to the location of the center.

Edgar Cayce's Vision of the Lord's Prayer & the Spiritual Centers of the Body	
Prayer/**Key Word**	Order/Gland/Center
Our Father/Mother which art in **Heaven**	7th/Pituitary/Third Eye
hallowed be thy **Name**	6th/Pineal/Crown
Thy kingdom come, thy **Will**	5th/Thyroid/Throat
be done; in **Heaven,** so in **Earth.**	(Heaven represents the three upper centers, earth the four lower ones.)
Give us for tomorrow the **Bodily Needs**	1st/Ovaries-Testes/ Root
And forgive us our **Trespasses**	3rd/Adrenals/Solar Plexus
as we forgive those who have and do trespass against us. And be thou the **Guide**	2nd/Leydig/Lyden ("the seat of the soul")
in the times of turmoil, temptation, and trouble; leading us through paths of **Righteousness—**	4th/Thymus/Heart
right heart, right attitude, right purposes; for Thy **Name's sake.**	6th/Pineal/Crown

To fully realize the power of this prayer, one must understand that it is intended to call forth the highest in each center. Just as we felt the words *still* and *God* in the earlier affirmation/mantra, so now we must feel or imagine the change brought on by these words and their meanings. Take your time. Consider this as part of the meditation period.

The order of the spiritual-centers prayer is significant in that it attempts to awaken the higher centers before awakening the lower ones. This is the best approach. Awakening the first center before the seventh and sixth is like opening the serpent basket without the charm of the flute. The serpent is loose to its own interests, rather than under the charm of the higher music. Keep a higher ideal, a higher purpose, a right heart, and the consciousness focused predominantly on the higher centers. Draw the kundalini upward.

BREATH POWER

Now once again we take hold of the breath. This time we take a stronger hold and use it in ways that arouse the life force and draw it up through the centers of this wonderful biospiritual instrument in which we abide. Why the breath? Cayce answers:

"BREATH is the basis of the living organism's activity. This opening of the centers or the raising of the life force may be brought about by certain characters of breathing—for, as indicated, the breath is power in itself; and this power may be directed." 2475-1

STRENGTHENING AND OPENING BREATH

There are several breathing patterns we could use. I'll focus on the ones that, in my experience, work best. The first is described often in Cayce's discourses. It begins with a deep inhalation through the right nostril, filling the lungs and feeling *strength!* Then exhalation through the mouth. This should be felt throughout the torso of the body—STRENGTH! After three of these, shift to inhaling through the left nostril and exhaling through the right (not through the mouth). This time feel the opening of your centers. As you do this left-right nostril breathing, keep your focus on the third eye and crown centers, letting the other centers open toward these two. This will not be difficult because the sixth and seventh centers have a natural magnetism—just as the snake charmer's music.

When you have finished this breathing pattern, go through the prayer again slowly, directing your attention to each center as you recite the phrase and key word.

RISING AND DESCENDING BREATH

Then, begin the second breathing pattern. It goes like this: Breathe through your nostrils in a normal manner; however, with each inhalation feel or *imagine* the life force being drawn up from the lower centers to the crown of the head and over to the third-eye center. Hold the breath slightly, and then as you exhale, feel or imagine the life force bathing the centers as the energy descends through each, to the lowest center. Pause, then inhale while again feeling or imagining the drawing upward. Repeat this cycle about seven times at a comfortable pace—using your consciousness and breath to direct the movement in synchronization with the inhalations and exhalations. As the breath and life force rise, feel or imagine how they are cleansed and purified by the higher centers. As they descend, feel how they bathe the centers with this purified energy. Take your time, consider this as part of the meditation. Do about seven cycles of inhalations and exhalations.

"These exercises [yoga breathing] are excellent. Thus an entity puts itself, through such an activity [yoga breathing], into association or in conjunction with all it has EVER been or may be. For it loosens the physical consciousness to the universal consciousness. Thus ye may constructively use that ability of spiritual attunement, which is the birthright of each soul; ye may use it as a helpful influence in thy experiences in the earth." (2475-1)

THE RISING INCANTATION

After this rising breathing pattern, it is a good time to use a rising incantation. Take a deep breath, then as you very slowly exhale, direct your consciousness to the lowest chakra and begin moving the life force upward as you chant in a drone: "ah ah ah ah ah, a a a a a, e e e e e, i i i i i, o o o o o, u u u u u, m m m m m." Each sound is associated with a center. "Ah" with the first center (2072-10 states, "This is not R, but Ah," as the "a" in spa). "A" with the second center (sounds like long "a" in able). "E" with the solar plexus (sounds like long "e" in eve). "I" with the heart (a long "i" as in high). "O" with the throat (long "o" as in open). "U" with the pineal (sounds like the "u" in true) . And ending the chant with a long toning of "m" at the third eye center (like humming the "m" in room).

Remember that true incantation is an *inner sounding* which vibrates, stimulates and lifts the life force. It is done in a droning manner, with a monotonous, humming tone—vibrating the vocal cords and then directing this vibration to the centers, thus vibrating them. Feel the glands being tuned to the specific sound/vibration, and then carry your consciousness upward as the sound changes. Do this chanting three or more times, or until you feel its effect. You may also want to finish this chanting portion of the practice with a few soundings of the great OM chant (as in "home").

Often at this point in the meditation, the head will be drawn back, the forehead and crown may have pronounced sensations or vibrations, and the upper body and head may be moving back and forth, or side to side, or in a circular motion (circular is preferable). These are all natural results of the practice. In The Revelation, St. John associates body shaking ("earthquakes") with the opening of the sixth center, followed by "silence in heaven" as the seventh center opens.

INTO THE MIND

Now we want to move in consciousness, so let the breathing and body go on autopilot (the autonomic system will watch over them). You'll be semiconscious of the body from here on in the meditation.

At this point in the practice, the whole of the body, mind, and soul are aroused and alert. Now, the ideal held is the *formative influence*, and development proceeds according to the ideal held.

The mind has a somewhat different experience in this type of meditation than in the Magic Silence method. All self-initiated activity is suspended. The mind has been changing as we have raised the energies of the body. By now it is very still, yet quite alert. Stay here. Do not draw away or attempt to affect anything. Heightened expectancy and alertness is an excellent state of mind at this point. Here's where we have the greatest opportunity to receive God. Completely open your consciousness to God's. St. John says that he was "in the spirit" (this was John's way of saying that he was in meditation) and he "turned" (in consciousness) and his revelation began. St. John's word "turned" so precisely describes the cessation of all self-initiated activity. We too must reach a point in the meditation where we turn around from our constant outer-directed thought stream, becoming transfixed on God's consciousness, and purely receptive.

EXPANSION AND THE IMAGINATIVE FORCES

Cayce says that we should have a strong sense of expansion and universalization while in this state. He also recommends that we *imagine* this expansion as we progress. The imaginative forces should be used to help us reach higher consciousness. So, *imagine* expansion as you raise the life force in the early stages of the practice. According to Cayce, the pineal's primary function is "the impulse or imaginative" force (294-141). It is this center that aids in the transition from material consciousness to spiritual consciousness. Use your imaginative forces to aid in this transition. Also, Cayce adds, "Keep the pineal gland operating and you won't grow old—you will always be young!" (294-141) Again we see the rejuvenative powers of this stimulation.

A MORE WONDERFUL LIFE

The power gained from this type of meditation is not used to rule but to allow more of God's influence to come into our lives and into this dimension. We are the channels of God in this realm, if we choose to be so. We could literally transform this realm if more of us developed ourselves to be better, clearer channels of the Life Force, the Great Spirit, God. The residual effect of this is that our individual lives become more fulfilling, abundant, and rejuvenated. As Cayce often said, "In the doing comes the understanding"—not in the talking, the

reading, the believing, the knowing, or thinking—
but in the doing. So come on, take up your practice.
Not just to feel better, but that the Infinite may
manifest in the finite, lifting all to a more wonderful
life!